*Patient Care
Guidelines
for the EMT*

Patient Care Guidelines for the EMT

DISCARDED

Susan K. Damon, R.N., B.S.

Judith Reid Graves, R.N., M.A., EMT-P

A BRADY BOOK
PRENTICE HALL BUILDING
Englewood Cliffs, New Jersey 07632

Library of Congress Cataloging-in-Publication Data

Damon, Susan K.
  Patient care guidelines for the EMT / by Susan K. Damon and Judith Reid Graves.
    p.   cm.
  ISBN 0-89303-749-4
  1. Emergency medicine—Handbooks, manuals, etc. 2. Emergency medical technicians—Handbooks, manuals, etc. I. Graves, Judith Reid. II. Title.
  [DNLM: 1. Allied Health Personnel. 2. Emergencies. WX 215 D163p]
  RC86.8.D36 1989
  616'.025—dc19
  DNLM/DLC
  for Library of Congress   88-38297
                                                                 CIP

NOTICE: It is the intent of the authors and publisher that this manual be used as part of an EMT Basic course taught by a qualified instructor or by a certified EMT Basic. The care procedures presented here represent accepted practices in the United States. They are not offered as a standard of care. Prehospital level emergency care is to be performed under the authority and guidance of a licensed physician. It is the reader's responsibility to know and follow local care protocols as provided by the medical advisors directing the system to which he or she belongs. Also, it is the reader's responsibility to stay informed of emergency care procedure changes.

Editorial/production supervision and
  interior design: Lillian Glennon
Cover design: Ben Santora
Manufacturing buyer: Robert Anderson

© 1989 by Prentice-Hall, Inc.
A Division of Simon & Schuster
Englewood Cliffs, New Jersey 07632

All rights reserved. No part of this book may be
reproduced, in any form or by any means,
without permission in writing from the publisher.

Printed in the United States of America
10 9 8 7 6 5 4 3 2 1

0-89303-749-4

Prentice-Hall International (UK) Limited, *London*
Prentice-Hall of Australia Pty. Limited, *Sydney*
Prentice-Hall Canada Inc., *Toronto*
Prentice-Hall Hispanoamericana, S.A., *Mexico*
Prentice-Hall of India Private Limited, *New Delhi*
Prentice-Hall of Japan, Inc., *Tokyo*
Simon & Schuster Asia Pte. Ltd., *Singapore*
Editora Prentice-Hall do Brasil, Ltda., *Rio de Janeiro*

Contents

ACKNOWLEDGMENTS	*ix*
A MEDICAL DIRECTOR'S FOREWORD	*xi*
AN ADMINISTRATOR'S FOREWORD	*xiii*
BASIC EMERGENCY PATIENT CARE SKILLS	*1*

Assessing a Patient   1
  Initial Approach, 1
  Primary Survey, 1
  Secondary Survey, 2

Taking a Medical History   4
  Medical Illness, 4
  Traumatic Injuries, 4
  Special Considerations, 4

Neurological Assessment   5
  Vital Signs, 5
  Level of Consciousness, 6
  Eyes, 7
  Movement and Sensation, 7
  Special Considerations, 7

Primary EMT Skills   8
  Airway Maintenance and Oxygen Therapy, 8
  Airway Obstruction: Unconscious, 9

Airway Obstruction: Conscious, 10
CPR (One-Person), 11
Control of Bleeding: External, 12
Control of Bleeding: Internal, 13
Managing Shock, 13
Dressings and Bandaging, 14
Splinting Techniques, 15
Traction Splinting, 15
Extrication, 16
Patient Movement, 17
Spinal Immobilization, 17
Patient Positioning during Transport, 18
Triage, 18

PATIENT CARE GUIDELINES 20

Cardiac Emergencies 20
   Nontraumatic Cardiac Arrest; Sudden Cardiac Death, 20
   Acute Myocardial Infarction, 23
   Angina, 24
   Congestive Heart Failure, 26

Environmental Emergencies 28
   Bites and Stings, 28
   Burns, 30
   Cold-Related Injuries, 32
   Drowning and Near-Drowning, 35
   Heat-Related Injuries, 37
   Inhalation Injuries, 39
   Mountain Sickness, 41
   Scuba Diving Accidents, 42

Medical Emergencies 45
   Abdominal Pain, 45
   Alcohol-Related Emergencies, 47
   Aneurysms (Thoracic and Abdominal), 49
   Behavioral Emergencies, 51
   Coma, 53
   Diabetic Emergencies, 55
   Drug Abuse and Overdose, 57
   Hypertensive Emergencies, 60
   Seizures, 62
   Stroke (CVA), 64

Obstetrical Emergencies 66
   Emergency Normal Childbirth, 66
   Prepartum Hemorrhage, 69

Breech Delivery, 70
Prolapsed Cord, 71
Cord around the Neck, 72
Postpartum Hemorrhage, 72
Premature Birth, 73
Multiple Births, 74
Spontaneous Abortion, 75
Ectopic Pregnancy, 76
Toxemia, 77
Toxic Shock Syndrome, 78
Rape and Sexual Assault, 79

Pediatric Emergencies   80
  Apnea, 80
  Child Abuse, 80
  Croup, 83
  Dehydration and Hypovolemia, 84
  Epiglottitis, 85
  Febrile Seizures, 86
  Poisonings, 87
  Sudden Infant Death Syndrome, 89

Respiratory Emergencies   90
  Asthma, 90
  Chronic Obstructive Pulmonary Disease, 91
  Hyperventilation Syndrome, 93
  Pneumonia, 94
  Pneumothorax (spontaneous), 95
  Pulmonary Edema, 96
  Pulmonary Embolism, 97
  Respiratory Distress, 98

Shock   100
  General Protocols for Shock, 100
  Anaphylactic Shock, 102
  Cardiogenic Shock, 103
  Hypovolemic Shock, 104
  Neurogenic Shock, 106
  Respiratory Shock, 107
  Septic Shock, 108

Traumatic Injuries   108
  Traumatic Cardiopulmonary Arrest, 108
  Abdominal Trauma, 109
  Amputations, 111
  Chest Injuries, 112
  Facial Injuries, 115
  Fractures, Dislocations, and Sprains, 118

Head Injuries, 120
Femur Fractures, 122
Hip Injuries (High Femur) in the Elderly, 123
Hip Injuries (High Femur) in the Young, 124
Pelvic Injuries, 125
Spinal Cord Injuries, 127
Throat Injuries, 129

APPENDICES 131

Appendix 1: Bag-Valve-Mask (FATS) Technique   131
Appendix 2: Community Resources   132
Appendix 3: Conversion Tables   132
Appendix 4: Diabetic Coma and Shock Fact Sheet   133
Appendix 5: Drugs Commonly Prescribed   134
Appendix 6: Medical Antishock Trousers (MAST) Procedure   137
Appendix 7: Medical Incident Report Form; SOAP Reporting   138
Appendix 8: Medical Radio Report   140
Appendix 9: Mettag Use for Disasters   141
Appendix 10: Techniques of Helmet Removal   143
Appendix 11: Oxygen Administration   147
Appendix 12: Paramedic Request: When to Call for Advanced Help   147
Appendix 13: Postural Blood Pressure and Heart Rate   150
Appendix 14: Restraints for Aggressive or Violent Patients   152
Appendix 15: Vital Signs   152
Appendix 16: Emergency Intravenous Fluid Therapy   153
Appendix 17: Communicable Disease Prevention   153
Appendix 18: Syrup of Ipecac   170

Acknowledgments

The completion of a project of this magnitude and depth is possible only through the combined efforts of many different people. To these people we wish to extend a very special thanks:

Steven Call, Manager, King County EMS (KCEMS) Division, understood the need for EMTs to have a reliable reference available to help them in their efforts to provide safe and consistent high-quality patient care. He identified this as a priority project and extended the time and personnel necessary to do the job.

Richard Cummins, M.D., M.P.H., Medical Director of the King County EMT Defibrillation Program, being well experienced in working with EMTs and highly respected by them, provided excellent medical advice and guidance throughout this project.

Jane Blackstone, Assistant Manager, KCEMS Division, wrote the guidelines for communicable diseases to be consistent with recommendations of the Centers for Disease Control.

Gregg Berguist, Renton Fire Department; Barbara Danielson and Cindy Hambly, King County Fire District (KCFD) No. 47; William Flora, KCFD No. 25; Douglas Austin, K. C. EMT Program Coordinator; and Thomas Torell, K. C. EMT Training Coordinator, for their assistance and hard work in helping to write these guidelines.

In addition, we must also thank those EMTs and paramedics who met with us periodically to review the many drafts and to discuss specific problems regarding EMT practices and treatments relevant to the guidelines. Their suggestions and comments were invaluable.

A personal thanks from us to Dorothy Bay, who spent countless hours at the word processor editing and revising drafts too numerous to count.

And let us not forget Claire Merrick, the one person who, in her wisdom and foresight, saw the significance of patient care guidelines for the working EMTs around the nation.

Susan K. Damon
Judith Reid Graves

Medical Director's Foreword

In many systems emergency medical technicians work with little supervision or guidance. Treatment provided by the emergency medical technicians may be unknown or even unacceptable to paramedics and emergency room physicians. Medical control of basic life support services in the form of case-by-case care review is not practical in many systems. Textbooks on emergency care, while informative and useful, often end treatment recommendations with the advice: "See your local treatment protocols." Frequently, these "local treatment protocols" are nowhere to be found.

The EMT treatment guidelines in this book were developed to address these problems. These guidelines have four purposes:

1. To provide advice to EMTs for specific problems they encounter in the field
2. To coordinate patient care in a tiered emergency medical system that begins with the EMT, continues with the paramedic, and ends with the emergency room physician
3. To define the extent and limits of the care that EMTs can provide
4. To provide prospective medical control to EMT actions

These guidelines arose from a unique process. First, the major textbooks for emergency medical technicians were reviewed and their treatment guidelines summarized. Next, the guidelines were modified to reflect EMT training curricula of various states. Then a group of experienced EMT instructors and trainers were brought together to review the recommendations and make any necessary changes and qualifications. Finally, paramedics and paramedic medical directors were consulted. The paramedic medical directors represented the emergency room physicians, who must continue the care initiated in the field by EMTs. The paramedics and their medical directors were asked the simple question: "What should the EMTs have done prior to paramedics and emergency room physicians taking over the care of patients?"

There were prolonged discussions and even some disagreement over many topics. This reflects that there is "no one *best* way" to treat many of the problems that EMTs face in their practice. The process we followed assured general agreement of what constitutes proper and approved initial prehospital care. The value of these guidelines for initial instruction, continuing education, legal protection, and medical control are obvious.

Various EMS systems may change some of the details of the treatment guidelines to coincide with different local system variations. Future experience and new information may also dictate that some of these guidelines be changed.

We think that EMTs will find these guidelines valuable for review and as a basis for interacting with paramedics and emergency physicians. Best of all, we think they will help provide improved care for the community as a whole—and that is what prehospital emergency care is really all about.

Richard O. Cummins, M.D., M.P.H.

An Administrator's Foreword

Patient Care Guidelines for the EMT were developed as a treatment reference manual for EMTs. It is a guide to tell them what to do, not a rationale of why or a description of how to perform skills. It provides a systematic approach to address various emergency situations, and leaves an EMT free to consider the technical tasks at hand. These guidelines give an EMT a reasonable list of treatment tasks and define a performance expectation that becomes a base for evaluating prehospital care. This guide can be used to examine emergency interventions performed and documented by EMTs on their Medical Incident Report Forms.

We have intentionally used the term *guidelines* and avoided such terms as *protocols, regulations,* or *standards*. The term *protocol* implies a rigid, inflexible approach to patient care. A "cookbook" approach to EMT field performance ignores the adverse environment in which an EMT performs his or her skills. These guidelines help define the kind of care expected to be provided for various emergency situations. (We acknowledge that these skills are often performed at night, in the rain, under a truck, with a Doberman barking at the EMT.) These are not formulas. They will not replace good judgment in a prehospital setting. They should be used as a supplement to the basic EMT textbook and enable the EMT to provide smooth emergency patient care while assessing the patient, establishing priorities, and executing the skills they were trained to perform.

Patient care guidelines have an important place in a medical care delivery system. They will complement training programs and instill confidence in EMTs, administrators, and medical directors. Use this guide to link all the interrelated elements of an EMS system together at the most important point of the system . . . the patient who desperately needs emergency medical treatment.

Steven Call, Manager
King County Emergency Medical Services Division

Patient Care Guidelines for the EMT

Basic Emergency Patient Care Skills

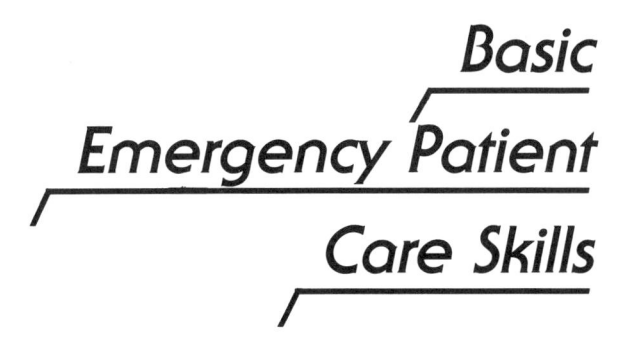

ASSESSING A PATIENT

Initial Approach

1. Inspect patient surroundings and identify environmental hazards.
2. Initiate communication and call for backup help if appropriate.
3. Identify number of patients and triage.
4. Identify and correct any life-threatening problems.
5. Identify mechanism of injury.
6. Introduce self to patient; reassure patient and request permission to treat.
7. Ask for patient's name and age.
8. Ask for patient's chief complaint.

Primary Survey

1. *Airway:* Open; look, listen, and feel; treat for any airway obstruction found.
2. *Breathing:* Note rate, effort, and abnormal sounds; observe skin color.
3. *Circulation:* Note presence and quality of pulse.

4. *Bleeding:* Stop major bleeding; observe for signs of shock: cool, clammy, pale skin; weak and fast pulse.
5. *Level of consciousness:* conscious, altered consciousness, or unconscious.
6. *Initial vital signs:* Pulse, respiratory rate, and blood pressure.

Note: Assume a cervical spine injury in any patient with injury above the level of the clavicles or anytime the mechanism of injury is sufficient to cause spinal injury (do this even in the absence of significant physical findings). Special attention is directed toward stabilizing the neck when establishing the airway using chin lift or jaw thrust maneuvers. The neck must be stabilized by one EMT while a second EMT completes the primary survey, and then a semirigid cervical collar should be applied. For further spinal immobilization techniques, see page 17.

Secondary Survey

This is a quick head-to-toe examination.

1. *Head and face*
   a. Gently palpate for depressions of skull and matted hair on the scalp.
   b. Observe for facial symmetry; palpate facial bones.
   c. *Eyes:* Are pupils equal and reactive to light? Check for foreign bodies, contact lenses, lacerations, and evidence of trauma and alterations in vision.
   d. *Ears:* Bleeding or fluid.
   e. *Nose:* Deformity, discharge, bleeding.
   f. *Mouth:* Dentures, loose, chipped, or avulsed teeth; tongue; foreign objects.
2. *Neck:* Evaluate front and back of neck unless done during the primary survey on trauma patients. Look for neck vein distension, stomas, use of neck muscles for respirations, altered voice, tracheal shift, or bruising.
3. *Spine and back:* Palpate skin for wounds, deformities, tenderness, or possible fractures starting from shoulders working toward buttocks.
4. *Chest*
   a. Auscultate for breath sounds.
   b. Palpate clavicles.

c. Observe for equal chest expansion on both sides.
   d. Gently press on lateral ribs to check for fractures.
   e. Gently perform rib spring on sternum to check for pain.
5. *Abdomen*
   a. Inspect for wounds, evisceration, distension, and scars.
   b. Gently palpate for rigidity, tenderness, guarding, and pulsating masses.
6. *Pelvis, hips, and buttocks*
   a. Palpate both sides for wounds, fractures, and tenderness.
   b. Check for distal pulses, sensation, and color.
7. *Shoulders/upper extremities*
   a. Palpate both sides for wounds, possible fractures, and tenderness.
   b. Check for distal pulses, sensation, color, and needle marks.
   c. Check for weakness by having the patient squeeze your hands if no obvious fracture present.
8. *Lower extremities*
   a. Palpate for wounds, possible fractures, deformities, tenderness, and skin discoloration.
   b. Check for distal pulses, capillary refill, sensation, and movement.
   c. Check for weakness by having the patient push with foot against your hand if no obvious fracture present.
9. *Vital signs*
   a. Obtain second full set of vital signs after secondary survey, including an auscultated blood pressure, pulse, respirations, pupillary reaction, skin temperature and color, and level of consciousness.
   b. Repeat according to patient's condition, or at least one more set prior to transport or enroute.
   c. Obtain postural blood pressure *in medical emergencies only* (see Appendix 13). Indications for checking postural BP:
      (1) Patient complains of lightheadedness or dizziness.
      (2) Patient complains of generalized weakness without apparent reason.
      (3) Patient who appears stable but has nonspecific complaints of illness.
   d. Monitor vital signs every 5 minutes during transport; record any changes.

TAKING A MEDICAL HISTORY

Medical Illness

1. Chief complaint
   a. Onset (When did this episode begin?)
   b. Character/nature of complaint
   c. Severity
   d. Duration
   e. Relief/aggravation
   f. Associated symptoms
   g. Location and/or radiation of pain
2. Other complaints
3. Related medical history
4. Allergies/medical alert information
5. Medications and drugs
6. Private physician

Traumatic Injuries

1. *Mechanism of injury:* type of accident and the expected injuries
   a. *Accidents:* motor vehicles, falls, gunshot wounds, fires, explosions, toxic inhalations, machinery, electrical shocks, swimming, boating, driving
   b. *Types of injuries:* soft tissue injuries, fractures, dislocations, internal injuries
2. *Patient complaint*
   a. Do you have any difficulty breathing?
   b. Do you hurt anywhere?
   c. What happened?
3. *Relevant medical history*
4. *Allergies/medical alert tag*
5. *Medications and drugs*
6. *Private physician*

Special Considerations

1. A patient's history is often obtained while performing the secondary survey. More information may be gathered from relatives or bystanders.
2. Information about the physical surroundings and environment can be invaluable to understanding the patient's condition and should be included in all reports.

3. When evaluating single-person accidents, consider an underlying medical cause of trauma.
4. The following questions will assist the EMT in obtaining the history of patients with complaints of medical illness:
   a. Describe for me what happened.
   b. Has this ever happened before? If yes, what did you (the patient) do about it then?
   c. When did it start?
   d. What were you doing when it started?
   e. Does anything make it better or worse?
   f. What have you done for the problem so far? Have you taken any medicine(s) for this problem? If yes, what medicine, how much, and when?
   g. Do you have any other current medical problems?
   h. Do you take any other medicine(s)?
   i. *If the complaint is about pain:*
      (1) Have patient point to the affected area.
      (2) Have patient describe the nature of the pain (i.e., sharp, dull, steady, cramping, pressure, intermittent).
      (3) Have patient describe the level of pain now compared to when it was most intense.

NEUROLOGICAL ASSESSMENT

Managing patients with head injuries or neurological illnesses depends on careful evaluation and observation of neurogenic function. These first observations made by EMTs in the field are crucial to establishing a baseline for monitoring and evaluating changes in a patient's condition. By providing an accurate baseline, the hospital staff is better able to decide whether to operate immediately.

The following are important observations to be made as part of the neurological assessment in the field. This information must be reported at the time the patient is transferred to another health care provider, and recorded in a written report.

Vital Signs

1. *Pulse and blood pressure*
   a. A rising blood pressure and a falling pulse may indicate that pressure inside the skull is rising as a result of bleeding within the skull or swelling of the brain (cerebral edema).

b. Hypovolemic shock is usually not the result of an isolated head injury, so look for other signs of internal or external bleeding.
2. *Respirations:* Look for changing patterns or respirations that become labored, then rapid, then stop for a few seconds.

Level of Consciousness

The single most important sign in evaluating a head injury is a changing level of consciousness. Coma scales can be useful in communicating a patient's level of consciousness. AVPU is a quick way to compile the patient's level of consciousness:

A (alert)
V (responsive to voice)
P (responsive to pain)
U (Unresponsive)

The Glasgow Coma Scale is a means of measuring and monitoring a patient's level of consciousness by calculating a score based on the best verbal, motor, and eye response. The lowest score possible is 3 and the highest is 15.

Best Verbal Response

Oriented and talking	5
Disoriented and confused	4
Inappropriate words	3
Incomprehensible	2
No response	1

Best Motor Response

Obeys commands	6
Locates pain	5
Withdraws from pain	4
Flexes to pain	3
Extends to pain	2
No response	1

Eye Response

Opens spontaneously	4
Opens to voice	3
Opens to pain	2
No response	1

Eyes

1. Note direction of gaze.
   a. Eyes gazing left or right
   b. Gaze conjugate or dysconjugate
2. Note size and reaction of pupils to light.
   a. Unequal or unresponsive
3. Note vision impairment.
4. Note evidence of trauma.

Movement and Sensation

1. Note movement of all extremities.
2. Note absent, abnormal, or normal sensation.
3. Note abnormal posturing.

Special Considerations

1. Signs and symptoms of brain injury can be similar to the signs and symptoms exhibited by a patient intoxicated or on drugs. Do not assume intoxication or drug abuse.
2. If an unconscious patient regains consciousness or lapses back into unconsciousness, this is a significant sign that must be reported. Any change in level of consciousness is a significant sign.
3. Any patient with head or face injury is assumed to have neck and spinal injuries and is treated as such.
4. When eliciting the best motor response, note the type of stimulus used. If a mild stimulus such as a light pinch or dull pinprick is unsuccessful, try pressure with a dull object to the base of the nailbed, a stronger pinch at the axilla.
5. Combative behavior is frequently a sign of head injury or of lack of oxygen to the brain.

PRIMARY EMT SKILLS

Airway Maintenance and Oxygen Therapy

1. Open airway using head-tilt, chin-lift, or modified jaw-thrust technique.
2. Insert oropharyngeal airway on unconscious patient with absent gag reflex only (use on semiconscious or conscious patients may cause vomiting or spasm of the vocal cords).
    a. Choose correct size by measuring from the corner of the mouth to ear lobe.
    b. Open the patient's mouth using the cross-finger technique.
    c. Insert airway with the tip facing upward toward the roof of the patient's mouth.
    d. When halfway in, rotate airway 180° and insert until the flange rests on the lips or teeth.
3. Administer oxygen.
    a. *Conscious patient:* Begin with 2 liters per minute (LPM) by cannula until history obtained.
    b. *COPD patient:* Provide 2 LPM by cannula or 24 percent by venturi mask unless in severe respiratory distress, when a moderate to high flow of oxygen may be indicated.
    c. *Cardiac and respiratory arrest:* Perform ventilation by bag-valve-mask with oxygen reservoir to deliver 100 percent.
    d. Impairment of respiratory or cardiovascular function (shock, bleeding, trauma, angina, myocardial infarction, head injuries, respiratory distress) requires 100 percent oxygen at high flow by face mask, or partial or full nonrebreathing mask.
    e. Oxygen flow rates:
       (1) Low flow   2–4 LPM   Nasal cannula
       (2) Moderate flow   5–9 LPM   Cannula, face mask, or partial rebreathing mask (6 LPM is maximum flow for cannula; minimum flow for mask)
       (3) High flow   10–15 LPM Nonrebreathing mask or bag-valve device with reservoir for 100 percent
4. Suction as needed.
    a. Insert suction catheter (preferably the Yankauer device)

Airway Obstruction: Unconscious

	Infant, Child, and Adult	Infant (0–12 Months)	Child (1–8 Years)	Adult
1.	Determine unresponsiveness, call for help, position the victim; open the airway, determine breathlessness.			
2.	Attempt ventilation; if unsuccessful, reposition and try again.			
3.		a. Deliver 4 blows between the shoulder blades. b. Deliver 4 chest thrusts in the midsternal region in the same manner as external chest compressions but at a slower rate (3–5 sec).	Perform 6–10 abdominal thrusts.	Perform 6–10 abdominal thrusts.
4.		Perform tongue–jaw lift. Do not perform blind finger sweep; remove foreign body only if visible.	Perform tongue–jaw lift. Do not perform blind finger sweep; remove foreign body only if visible.	Perform deep finger sweep into mouth to remove foreign body.
5.	Reattempt ventilation			
6.	Repeat sequence until obstruction relieved.			

Airway Obstruction: Conscious

Infant, Child, and Adult	Infant (0–12 Months)	Child (1–8 Years)	Adult
1.	Determine obstruction by observing for breathing difficulties.[a]	Determine if victim can cough or speak.	Determine if victim can cough or speak.
2.	Deliver 4 chest thrusts.	Perform abdominal thrusts if victim's cough is ineffective and victim is experiencing respiratory difficulty.	Perform abdominal thrusts if victim's cough is ineffective and victim is experiencing respiratory difficulty.
3. Repeat sequence above until either foreign body is expelled or victim becomes unconscious.			

[a] This procedure should be evaluated in a conscious infant only if the airway obstruction is due to a witnessed or strongly suspected aspiration and if respiratory difficulty is increasing and cough is ineffective. If obstruction is caused by airway swelling due to infection (epiglottis or croup), these procedures may be harmful. Paramedics should be requested or the infant transported immediately.

CPR (One-Person)

Infant, Child, and Adult	Infant (0–12 Months)	Child (1–8 Years)	Adult
1. Determine unresponsiveness, position the victim.			
2. Open airway.	Head tilt/chin lift maneuver to sniffing or neutral position.	Use head tilt/chin lift maneuver.	Use head tilt/chin lift maneuver.
3. Determine breathlessness.	3–5 sec	3–5 sec	3–5 sec
4. Ventilate 2 times (1–1.5 sec per ventilation) using breaths to make chest rise.	Small breaths		
5. Determine pulselessness.	Palpate brachial pulse.	Palpate carotid pulse.	Palpate carotid pulse.
6. Begin chest compressions.	Rate: 100/min (5 compressions/3 sec or less).	Rate: 80–100/min (5 compressions/3–4 sec).	Rate: 80–100/min (15 compressions/9–11 sec).
7. Compression/ventilation ratio. Check pulse to assess compressions.	5:1	5:1	15:2
8. Reassessment.	Palpate brachial pulse. Resume CPR if no pulse.	Palpate carotid pulse and resume CPR if no pulse.	Palpate carotid pulse and resume CPR if no pulse.
9. Resume compression/ventilation cycles.	Ventilate once, then begin compressions.	Ventilate once, then begin compressions.	Ventilate twice, then compressions.

into pharynx; length of insertion is the measured distance from mouth to lobe of ear.
b. Apply suction only after catheter in place.
c. Suctioning should not exceed 15 seconds.
d. Ensure adequate ventilation and oxygenation between suctioning.
e. In many instances, suction devices may be inadequate and the patient may have to be positioned on either side to facilitate clearing the airway.
f. When transporting a patient, suction apparatus should be assembled, turned on, and placed near the head for ready use.
5. Monitor adequacy of ventilation and oxygenation during all patient care.
6. Choose correct equipment and technique to assist in ventilations if necessary.
a. For one-person CPR, the pocket-face mask is more appropriate.
b. For two-person CPR, the bag-valve-mask and FATS (face and thigh smash) technique is more appropriate (see Appendix 1).

SPECIAL CONDITIONS

1. In instances other than cardiac arrest, CPR should be initiated when the following conditions exist:
a. Unconsciousness
b. Systolic blood pressure less than or equal to 60 mmHg
2. Personal preference by medics—stopping compression for intubations as directed by paramedics.

Control of Bleeding: External

1. Apply direct pressure to the open wound by placing gauze or clean material against the bleeding point and apply pressure.
2. Additional pressure should be applied with the other hand if bleeding continues. Pressure dressing, BP cuff, or air splint can also be used to apply direct pressure.
3. If not contraindicated by the injury, elevate the bleeding extremity above the level of the heart.

4. If bleeding is uncontrolled with direct pressure and elevation, pressure should be applied at the appropriate pressure point (indirect pressure).
   a. Pressure points are used only after direct pressure fails, and done so cautiously since damage can result from inadequate blood flow.
   b. Indirect pressure should be held only as long as necessary to control bleeding, and should be reapplied if bleeding recurs.
5. Consider use of the antishock trousers to control external or internal bleeding of the extremities or abdomen.

Control of Bleeding: Internal

1. Administer high concentration of oxygen by mask.
2. If internal bleeding is suspected in abdomen, pelvis, or legs, apply and inflate the antishock trousers (see Appendix 6 for the MAST procedure).
3. Application of a splint may help to control internal bleeding suspected on a fractured extremity.
4. Monitor and treat for shock.
5. Transport immediately.

Managing Shock

1. Maintain open airway. Assist respirations as needed.
2. Administer high flow (10 to 15 LPM) of 100 percent oxygen by nonrebreather mask or bag-valve-mask device.
3. Control obvious bleeding.
4. Splint all fractures.
5. If systolic BP below 90 and pulse rate above 110, or SBP below 80 regardless of pulse, apply and inflate medical antishock trousers if available.
6. If MAST unavailable, lay patient flat and elevate legs 30° or 12 inches.
7. If patient is immobilized on a backboard, elevate lower end of board 30° or 12 inches.
8. Keep the patient warm.
9. Transport the patient to a hospital as soon as possible.
10. Start IV with large-bore needle enroute.

11. Apply ECG monitor leads for patient with medical emergencies.
12. Manage all types of shock as described, with the exception of the following:
    a. *Anaphylactic shock:* Assist the person, if conscious and alert, in administering injectable or oral antiallergenic medication.
    b. *Neurogenic shock:* Stabilize neck and immobilize on long backboard.
    c. *Cardiogenic shock:* Use of the medical antishock trousers is absolutely contraindicated.
13. Cover patient to avoid excess heat loss, but do not overwrap.
14. Keep patient warm and off the ground; move out of the weather.
15. Give nothing by mouth.
16. Have suction available.
17. Monitor vital signs and level of consciousness.
18. If paramedics are available, transport to a hospital immediately.

Dressings and Bandaging

1. Control bleeding.
2. Use sterile or very clean materials.
3. Dress the entire wound.
4. Do not remove dressing once applied. If bleeding continues, add new dressings over blood-soaked ones.
5. Secure dressing with bandage that is snug but does not impair circulation. Check for presence of pulses distal to bandages.
6. Remove loose ends that might get caught on objects as the patient is moved.
7. Leave uncovered tips of fingers and toes so that skin color changes can be observed.
8. Bandage body part in the position it is to be left, since swelling frequently follows an injury.
9. Preserve avulsed and amputated parts. Severed parts should be saved and flaps of skin may be folded back to their normal position before bandaging. All severed parts and fragments (bone chips, teeth, fingers, toes, etc.) should be wrapped in a sterile dressing, placed in a zip-lock bag or container, and put on ice.

10. Do not remove impaled objects, but secure in place and bandage. *Exception:* Remove impaled object in the cheek and pack with dressings to protect airway from bleeding.
11. Do not replace protruding organs. As with eviscerated abdominal contents, apply a sheet of sterile saran wrap followed by a bulky, dry dressing. Do not moisten the dressing.
12. Elevate injured extremity when possible to decrease swelling in the injured area.

Splinting Techniques

1. Remove or cut away clothing.
2. Cover all wounds with a sterile dressing.
3. Check pulse and neurological status distal to injury before moving.
4. Do not replace protruding bones; may reduce with traction splinting.
5. For treatment of fractures, dislocations, and sprains, see page 118.
6. Consider use of medical antishock trousers for complicated femur fractures or pelvic fractures (see Appendix 6).
7. Immobilize joint injuries in position found.
8. Immobilize the joint above and below the fracture or dislocation.
9. Pad and splint to prevent pressure points.
10. Splint all fractures *before* moving the patient.
11. Check distal pulses, motor function, and sensation before and after splinting, and leave pulse points open for assessing arterial blood flow. This is a true emergency when distal pulse is absent. Transport as soon as possible.
12. Splint whenever in doubt.
13. Elevate extremity after splinting. Place cold pack near site.
14. Transport as soon as possible.

Traction Splinting (Femur Fractures Only)

1. Remove or cut away clothing.
2. Control bleeding; cover all wounds with sterile dressing.
3. Check distal pulse, sensation, and movement before splinting.

4. Measure splint length prior to application; open and position the ischial pad and straps to be applied midthigh, above and below the knee, and above the ankle.
5. Wrap the ankle hitch around the patient's foot.
6. Apply manual traction to the ankle hitch and foot while supporting the limb.
7. Position the splint in place. Secure the groin strap first.
8. Support of the limb is released only after traction has been achieved and the ankle hitch has been secured.
9. Secure remaining straps.
10. Recheck distal pulse, sensation, and movement.
11. Apply ice or cold pack to affected area.
12. Elevate injured leg by raising splint stand.
13. Assume spinal injury with femur fractures, and treat appropriately.
14. Transport.
15. Start large-bore IV enroute.

Extrication

1. Evaluate and secure the scene.
   a. Survey for potential hazards.
   b. Note number of patients.
   c. Call for additional personnel and equipment.
   d. Provide traffic control.
2. Stabilize vehicle before entry.
3. Gain access to the victim(s). All steps involved with extrication must be done in a manner that minimizes any chances of further injury.
4. Complete primary survey on all patients before management.
5. Treat airway difficulties and severe bleeding first.
6. Apply steady, gentle traction to the head and neck while cervical collar is applied. Maintain manual traction until patient is secured to a backboard.
7. Perform secondary survey as quickly as possible; splint extremity fractures if possible before extricating.
8. Properly secure patient on short board or extrication device.
9. Protect patient during removal of dangerous objects such as broken glass and jagged metal.

10. Maintain head traction, spinal alignment, and immobilization of patient during extrication.
11. Complete secondary survey and secure patient onto long spine board using adequate padding and ties.

Patient Movement

1. All injured parts should be immobilized as much as possible prior to movement and before transport.
2. All injured parts should be protected during movement.
3. When treating suspected spinal injuries and backboard or clamshell is unavailable, log roll the patient as a unit with three rescuers, or use some type of long axis pull (i.e., the foot drag, shoulder drag, fireman's drag, etc.).

Spinal Immobilization

1. Apply gentle but firm support to patient's head.
2. Apply semirigid cervical collar of correct size for the patient.
3. Apply extrication device (i.e., the Kendrick or CID) if available.
4. Extricate patient while maintaining spinal alignment and traction on the head.
5. Place on long backboard.
6. If not using an extrication device, place horseshoe-shaped blanket, sandbags, IV bags, or the like around patient's head.
7. Provide adequate padding along patient's sides, between legs, behind small of the back, and all other spaces.
8. Immobilize the head with 2-inch adhesive tape or crevat across forehead.
9. *Do not use chin strap or tape on chin.*
10. Immobilize chest by crisscrossing over shoulders across chest to hips.
11. Immobilize pelvis either crisscrossing over or straight across. Do not put pressure over bladder or abdominal injuries.
12. Place one strap across thighs above knees.
13. Place one strap across lower extremities.
14. Place one strap across feet.
15. Check pulses, sensation, and movement of lower extremities.

16. Patient should be effectively immobilized to allow turning as a unit for airway control.
17. Continued monitoring of airway and vital signs.

Patient Positioning during Transport

Proper positioning of the patient prior to transport depends on the nature of the illness or injuries.

1. *Stable angina or acute myocardial infarction that is uncomplicated:* position of comfort or semireclining. Do not lay flat unless in shock (see item 5).
2. *Conscious in respiratory distress:* position of comfort with head of stretcher elevated or semireclining.
3. *Nontraumatic illness with altered consciousness or coma* (seizures, alcoholism, diabetic coma, drug overdose): well secured to long backboard and positioned on its side if necessary for airway maintenance.
4. *Traumatic injury with altered consciousness or coma:* securely immobilized on long spine board. Tilt board on its side if patient begins to vomit.
5. *Shock:* flat with legs or backboard elevated to 30° or 12 inches unless using antishock trousers.

Triage

1. Complete primary survey on all patients and quickly treat life-threatening injuries only (similar to basic trauma survey except brief and without tools; BP is not obtained when triaging).
   a. *Airway:* Open airway.
   b. *Shock:* Elevate extremities.
   c. *Hazards:* Move patients.
   d. *Do not begin CPR until triage is completed.*
2. EMT secures Mettag to patient.
   a. *In-field triaging:* EMT tags and prioritizes injuries.
   b. *Central triaging:* Patient is moved to triage area, where triage leader assigns priorities.
3. Priority categorizations:
   a. *Priority I:* immediate treatment (RED)
      (1) Obstructed airway

  (2) Sucking chest wounds
  (3) Hypovolemic shock
  (4) Arterial bleed
  (5) Serious psychological problems
  (6) Arm/leg amputation with hemorrhage
  (7) Second-degree burns over more than 25 percent of body
  (8) Third-degree burns over more than 25 percent of body or with respiratory involvement
 b. *Priority II:* delayed treatment (YELLOW)
  (1) Second- and third-degree burns over more than 25 percent
  (2) Major bone fractures
  (3) Chest/abdominal trauma
  (4) Major lacerations
  (5) Eye injuries
 c. *Priority III:* minimal treatment (GREEN)
  (1) Minor contusions, lacerations
  (2) Second-degree burns over more than 20 percent of body except burns of the face and hands (priority II)
 d. *Priority* 0: expectant (BLACK)
  (1) Cardiac arrest
  (2) Critical CNS and respiratory injuries
  (3) People who have received massive doses of radiation
4. Patients are moved to appropriate areas and treated.

Patient Care Guidelines

CARDIAC EMERGENCIES

Nontraumatic Cardiac Arrest; Sudden Cardiac Death

DESCRIPTION

Nontraumatic cardiac arrest occurs suddenly with no warning or symptoms for 1 to 2 hours before the event. The heart stops pumping blood, which causes pulse and blood pressure to be absent. This is the leading cause of death in people over the age of 40 in the United States. Most patients have undetected coronary artery disease and may have had symptoms of an acute myocardial infarction.

SIGNIFICANT PHYSICAL FINDINGS

1. Unresponsive
2. Absent normal respirations; agonal attempts to breathe may be present
3. No pulse
4. Seizures due to lack of oxygen to the brain

SIGNIFICANT HISTORY

Do *not* delay treatment to obtain a history.

1. Was the collapse witnessed by a bystander, and was bystander CPR begun?

2. Were there symptoms of an acute myocardial infarction prior to the collapse?
3. Is there relevant medical history?

PATIENT CARE

Initiate CPR until a defibrillator is available. If you are authorized, operate a defibrillator following the standing orders provided by the medical director for your program. These are standing orders that follow EMT defibrillation national standards as outlined by the National Council of State Emergency Medical Services Training Coordinators.

Using either an automated or manually operated defibrillator, shock only the ECG rhythm ventricular fibrillation (VF) repeatedly and as quickly as possible. Interrupt CPR for a minimum of time and do not neglect general patient care or safety.

ECG RHYTHM ASSESSMENT

Confirm that the patient's ECG rhythm is VF by:

1. Activate power and voice tape recorder. (If required, calibrate manual defibrillator to 1 cm.)
2. Attach monitor leads or defibrillator electrodes.

Automated Defibrillators	Manual Defibrillators
Clear patient of all physical contact with rescuers.	Gel the paddles.
Switch into automatic mode.	Charge to 200 joules.
Wait 15 seconds.	Start ECG paper recorder.
	Clear patient of all physical contact with rescuers.

TREATMENT

Give the ECG rhythm VF up to a total of six countershocks. Give up to three shocks in a row with no CPR between those shocks if VF persists.

Automated Defibrillators

1. Have the defibrillator evaluate the ECG rhythm and shock the patient up to three times in a row.
2. When a 15-second interval passes without a shock, switch out of automated assessment mode and administer CPR for 15 to 30 seconds.
3. Switch back to automated assessment and treat the patient with up to three more shocks in a row.

Manual Defibrillators

1. Give one shock and leave the paddles in place on the chest; recharge to 200 joules; reassess the rhythm.
2. If VF persists, give shock 2 and leave the paddles on the patient's chest: recharge to 200 joules and reassess the ECG rhythm.
3. If VF is found, give shock 3.
4. Perform CPR for 15 to 30 seconds and repeat steps 1 to 3 if the rhythm VF is still present or returns.

SPECIAL CONSIDERATIONS FOR EMT DEFIBRILLATION

1. If a patient responds to early defibrillation and regains a pulse, continue to support their respirations, take a blood pressure, and administer CPR for systolic blood pressure below 60.
2. Manual defibrillators must use monitor leads to assess the ECG rhythm, not "quick-look paddles."
3. Children under the age of 12 or those who weigh less than 90 pounds should not be defibrillated by EMTs.
4. EMTs must meet the following requirements to provide lifesaving defibrillatory shocks to their patients.
   a. Maintain certification as an EMT.
   b. Complete a state-approved training course for EMT defibrillation.
   c. Perform defibrillation according to standing orders provided by the physician medical director.
   d. Provide complete documentation of each case using a cas-

sette recorder capable of recording both voice and cardiac rhythm during the cardiac arrest.
e. Maintain the defibrillation skills through a formal continuing education program.

Acute Myocardial Infarction

DESCRIPTION

Acute myocardial infarction (commonly known as a heart attack) is a condition in which a portion of the heart muscle (myocardium) dies as a result of oxygen starvation. This occurs as a result of a narrowing or occlusion of the coronary artery which supplies the myocardium with blood.

SIGNIFICANT PHYSICAL FINDINGS

1. Rapid, irregular pulse
2. Low blood pressure
3. Profuse sweating (diaphoresis)
4. Difficulty breathing or SOB
5. Frightened appearance
6. Restlessness, anxiety, confusion
7. Pale, gray skin color
8. Nausea, vomiting
9. Incontinence of urine and stool

SIGNIFICANT HISTORY

1. *Pain:* chest pain, tightness, pressure, epigastric pain, indigestion, or heartburn; severe and intense, lasting more than 15 minutes and unchanging; usually not brought on by exertion and not relieved by rest or nitroglycerin; radiating to arms, neck, jaws, and back
2. *Associated symptoms:* shortness of breath, sweatiness, nausea, vomiting, feeling of impending doom, weakness, dizziness, lightheadedness, cold and clammy
3. *Medical history:* previous cardiac problems, risk factors, surgeries, hospitalizations
4. *Current medications*

PATIENT CARE

1. Administer moderate flow (5 to 9 LPM) of oxygen by cannula or face mask.
2. Position of comfort in semireclining position. Do not lay flat.
3. Loosen tight clothing.
4. Reassure patient.
5. Monitor vital signs often.
6. Apply ECG monitor (Special Consideration 1).
7. Restrict patient movement; lift the patient to the stretcher.
8. Consider starting an IV of D_5W at KVO (keep vein open) with microdrip administration tubing.
9. Consider if paramedic evaluation required; if paramedics unavailable, transport immediately.
10. Transport without lights or sirens as quickly as possible.

SPECIAL CONSIDERATIONS

1. If certified in defibrillation, attach leads and monitor cardiac rhythm.
2. A major factor in heart disease is sudden death, or cardiac arrest that occurs within 2 hours of the onset of symptoms.
3. Complications of an acute myocardial infarction are:
   a. Arrhythmias (disturbance in heart rate and rhythm)
   b. Cardiac arrest
   c. Ventricular fibrillation
   d. Congestive heart failure
   e. Cardiogenic shock
4. Patients with chest pain commonly deny that anything is seriously wrong, often using such phrases as "it's just a little pressure" or "It's hardly worth bothering about."

Angina

DESCRIPTION

Angina pectoris is chest pain that occurs due to inadequate supply of blood to the heart muscle. Pain is usually transitory and is brought on by exertion or stress, lasting less than 10 minutes and relieved by cessation of activity and rest.

SIGNIFICANT PHYSICAL FINDINGS

1. Mild respiratory distress; respiratory rate slightly increased
2. Normal to slightly elevated pulse rate, but normal ECG rhythm
3. Normal blood pressure

SIGNIFICANT HISTORY

1. Description of pain
   a. Onset with exertion; relieved with rest and nitroglycerin
   b. Feels like pressure or squeezing beneath the sternum
   c. Radiates to jaw and arms
   d. Lasts 3 to 10 minutes
   e. Different from previous episodes
2. How many nitroglycerin tablets taken; is this different from usual pattern?
3. Accompanying symptoms: nausea, anxiety, general weakness
4. Medical history: chronic angina, cardiac problems, hospitalizations, surgery
5. Current medications

PATIENT CARE

1. Administer moderate flow (5 to 9 LPM) of oxygen by cannula or face mask.
2. Place patient at rest.
3. Position of comfort or semireclining.
4. Assist patient in taking nitroglycerin if prescribed to patient. (This is based on how many already taken and how many usually taken. But not to exceed maximum number prescribed by physician.)
5. Reassure patient.
6. Monitor vital signs closely.
7. Apply ECG monitor leads (Special Consideration 2).
8. Consider starting an IV of D_5W with microdrip administration tubing at KVO.
9. Paramedic evaluation required; if paramedics unavailable, transport immediately.
10. Transport without lights and sirens.

SPECIAL CONSIDERATIONS

1. When a patient with chronic angina calls for help, this usually indicates something different or unusual is happening: the pain is unrelieved, it is more severe, and so on. It should be assumed that such patients are having a heart attack and are in need of hospital evaluation.
2. If certified in defibrillation, attach leads and monitor cardiac rhythm.

Congestive Heart Failure

DESCRIPTION

Congestive heart failure (CHF) is the failure of the heart to pump efficiently as a result of damage to or weakening of the heart muscle. This in turn leads to the accumulation of fluids in the lungs and/or body, depending on whether the right or left side of the heart (or both) is involved. Acute left-sided heart failure can result in fluid accumulation in the lungs known as pulmonary edema. Failure of the right side leads to fluid accumulation, most notably in the lower extremities and ankles, and tends to be chronic and not life threatening.

The most common cause of CHF is a myocardial infarction. Other causes include chronic or sustained hypertension, diseased heart valves, or obstructive pulmonary diseases. Onset of symptoms is usually gradual over 3 to 7 days, and can be mild or severe and life threatening.

SIGNIFICANT PHYSICAL FINDINGS

1. Rapid pulse (120 or above)
2. Rapid, shallow respirations greater than 30 per minute
3. Frothy pink sputum may be present
4. Cyanosis
5. Distended neck veins
6. Anxiety or confusion
7. Edema, especially lower extremities and ankles (can be a chronic condition)
8. Rales (wet lung sounds)
9. Blood pressure usually elevated
10. Needs to sit up to breathe
11. Cannot talk in long sentences

SIGNIFICANT HISTORY

1. Chief complaint: shortness of breath
2. Awakening from sleep because of difficulty breathing, needing to sleep with several pillows, sleeping upright in a chair
3. Worsening of a chronic condition (i.e., increased ankle swelling, progressive fatigue, dyspnea)
4. Medical history, past hospitalizations
5. Medications
6. Associate complaints include:
   a. Chest pain
   b. Tiring from breathing
   c. Needs to sit up to breathe

PATIENT CARE

1. Administer high flow (10 to 15 LPM) of oxygen by nonrebreathing mask unless history of COPD.
   a. For COPD patients, low flow (2 to 4 LPM) of oxygen by cannula is recommended to start.
   b. If in obvious respiratory distress (see Appendix 11), administer high flow (10 to 15 LPM) of oxygen by nonrebreathing mask.
   c. Observe patients with COPD on oxygen for decreasing respirations and assist as needed.
2. Place in a semireclining position or upright with legs dangling.
3. Apply ECG monitor (if EMT-D certified).
4. Consider an IV D_5W with microdrip tubing KVO (if IV certified).
5. Request paramedic evaluation if condition indicates (see Appendix 12).

SPECIAL CONSIDERATIONS

1. A sudden worsening of chronic CHF is most often caused by a myocardial infarction.
2. Pulmonary edema is the most serious manifestation of CHF.
3. Never withhold oxygen therapy from a patient in respiratory distress, even with a history of COPD. Prepare to assist if respirations become depressed.

4. Use of the medical antishock trousers is absolutely contraindicated for CHF or pulmonary edema.

ENVIRONMENTAL EMERGENCIES

Bites and Stings

DESCRIPTION

Animal bites, snakebites, insect stings, and spider bites from a variety of species can result in serious illness and injury. Animal bites from wild animals such as skunks, bats, racoons, and foxes pose the special risk of rabies. Bites or stings from snakes, insects, or spiders inject a poisonous venom into its victims, generally affecting the cardiovascular or neurological system. Individual reactions to venom vary greatly depending on the person's sensitivity. Rapid anaphylactic shock can occur from a severe allergic reaction. Five percent of the general population is allergic to the sting of wasps, bees, hornets, yellow jackets, and ants. Insect stings cause twice as many deaths as snakebites each year.

SIGNIFICANT PHYSICAL FINDINGS

Moderate Reactions

1. Hives
2. Noticeable stings or bites on the skin
3. Puncture marks of the forearms or legs
4. Localized pain or itching
5. Burning sensation at the site, followed by pain spreading throughout the limb
6. Swelling or blistering at the site
7. Muscle cramps, chest tightness, joint pain
8. Excessive salivation, profuse sweating

Severe Reactions

1. Weakness, collapse
2. Difficulty breathing and swallowing
3. Headache, dizziness

4. Nausea, vomiting
5. Anaphylactic shock: rapid, weak pulse, low blood pressure (below 90 systolic), swelling of the face and tongue, flushing around the face and chest
6. Unconsciousness
7. Constricted upper airway sounds
8. Abnormal pulse rate or rhythm

SIGNIFICANT HISTORY

1. Medical alert tag
2. Source and time of exposure
3. Previous allergic reactions
4. Surrounding circumstances (i.e., bizarre behavior exhibited by animal prior to bite, etc.)
5. Medical history; current medications

PATIENT CARE

1. Assist with administration of injectable or oral medication.
2. Keep patient calm.
3. Maintain airway. Assist respirations as needed.
4. Administer oxygen if condition warrants.
5. Treat for shock, conserve body heat.
6. Alert the base hospital to secure antivenom if available.
7. Scrape away stingers and venom sacs; do not pull out stingers.
8. Locate fang marks if snakebite and clean with antiseptic.
9. Apply a light constricting band to reduce venous flow for venomous snakebites 2 inches above and 2 inches below wound (but not above or below joints).
   a. The band should be loose enough to allow sliding a finger underneath.
   b. Check for presence of arterial pulse below band.
   c. Remove bands for 1 minute every 10 minutes and move slightly.
   d. Bands are not beneficial if applied more than 30 minutes after the bite.

10. Immobilize bitten extremity level with or below level of the heart.
11. Remove rings, bracelets, or other constricting items on bitten extremity.
12. Identify or bring along dead organism if it can be done safely.
13. Notify animal control if appropriate.
14. Request paramedic evaluation if condition indicates (see Appendix 12).

SPECIAL CONSIDERATION

Do not apply an ice bag or cold pack on snakebites since this can cause additional tissue damage. However, ice bags can be applied to insect bites to reduce pain and swelling.

Burns

DESCRIPTION

Burns can vary in seriousness depending on many factors. Often, unsuspected or potentially life threatening injuries go undetected unless these factors are considered. Before appropriate field care can be given, the EMT must assess the severity of the burn by considering the following:

1. Degree of burn
2. Location of burn
3. Accompanying complications
4. Presence of other illnesses or injuries
5. Age of the patient

SIGNIFICANT PHYSICAL FINDINGS

1. *Appearance of the burn*
   a. *First degree:* bright red
   b. *Second degree:* red or mottled (spotting) skin with blisters
   c. *Third degree:* blackened (charred), leathery, dry and white
   d. *Fourth degree:* charred surface, exposed muscle/bone
2. *Extent of the burns:* description of areas involved

3. *Evidence of respiratory involvement:* charring of the mouth and nasal hairs, eyebrows, sooty residue, dyspnea, cough, hoarseness
4. *Signs of shock:* altered consciousness; rapid, weak pulse; cool, clammy skin; low blood pressure
5. *Secondary trauma*

SIGNIFICANT HISTORY

1. Mechanism or source of burn
2. Time elapsed since burn
3. Was patient in a closed space with steam or smoke? For how long?
4. Loss of consciousness
5. Accompanying explosion or toxic fumes
6. Prior chronic illness, history of cardiac or pulmonary disease
7. Treatment the burn received prior to EMT's arrival

PATIENT CARE

1. Remove patient from burning source.
   a. Remove clothing unless it is embedded in the wound.
   b. Dilute and rinse chemicals with large amounts of water.
   c. Brush dry solids off patient.
2. Manage airway and assist respirations as needed.
3. Control bleeding.
4. Administer high flow (10 to 15 LPM) of oxygen if history or presence of respiratory distress indicates need.
5. Treat for shock and consider use of the medical antishock trousers as follows:
   a. If SBP is 80 mmHg or less, all chambers of MAST can be inflated.
   b. If SBP between 80 and 90 mmHg and pulse is above 110, do not inflate MAST chambers over second- and third-degree burn areas.
6. Cover burns with sterile (whenever possible) dressings or sheets to prevent more contamination and infection to wounds.

a. If hands or toes are burned, separate digits with sterile gauze pads.
   b. Cover to conserve body heat and keep patient warm.
7. Do not apply ointments, sprays, creams, or oils to burns.
8. Do not disturb blisters.
9. Do not apply ice to burn areas.
10. Remove rings, bracelets, and other constricting items.
11. Elevate affected extremity.
12. Paramedic evaluation required for the following:
    a. Facial burns
    b. Second- or third-degree burns
    c. Respiratory involvement
13. Transport to hospital with access to a burn center as soon as possible.
14. Give the patient nothing by mouth.
15. If transporting to a hospital more than 20 minutes away, consider starting an IV of normal saline or lactated Ringer's solution with a large-bore needle.

SPECIAL CONSIDERATIONS

1. Blood pressure can be taken on a burned extremity by first placing gauze over area to be covered by BP cuff.
2. Attempt to leave unbroken blisters intact.
3. Suspect airway burns in any head, facial, or neck burns or burns received in a closed place.
4. Consider carbon monoxide poisoning in all closed space burns. If suspected, administer 100 percent oxygen at high flow (10 to 15 LPM) through a nonrebreather mask.
5. Eye burns may require flushing with normal saline and then patching the eyelids closed.

Cold-Related Injuries

DESCRIPTION

Frostbite and hypothermia are the most serious injuries resulting from prolonged exposure to extreme cold. If an environment is too cold, body heat will be lost faster than it can be generated, leading to damage of exposed tissue or a general reduction or cessation of vital body functions. *Frostbite* occurs when localized cooling causes the tissue of exposed body parts to freeze. The ears, nose, hands, and feet are most commonly affected. *Hypothermia* occurs when the core temperature of the body (the internal organs of the trunk) falls below 35°C/95°F (normal: 37°C/98.6°F).

SIGNIFICANT PHYSICAL FINDINGS

FROSTBITE

1. *Skin color changes:* white to gray to bluish gray and appears waxy
2. *Loss of sensation:* affected area feels numb
3. *Skin texture:* as frostbite progresses, surface and underlying tissue hardens
4. *Rewarming:* onset of tingling, unresponsiveness, stinging, and throbbing pain to excrutiating pain and formation of blisters associated with deep frostbite

HYPOTHERMIA

1. Intense, uncontrollable shivering
2. Difficulty speaking
3. Coordination difficulties, staggering
4. Poor judgment, lethargy
5. Confusion, irrational behavior
6. Decreased pulse and respirations
7. Unconsciousness, throbbing
8. Irregular pulse rate
9. Unobtainable blood pressure
10. Ice-cold skin

SIGNIFICANT HISTORY

1. Length of exposure
2. Loss of consciousness
3. Was the patient wet?
4. Were any drugs or alcohol used?
5. Any thawing attempts or refreezing of affected parts?
6. Age of patient
7. History of illnesses, injuries
8. Current medications

PATIENT CARE

FROSTBITE

1. Protect the injured areas from pressure, trauma, and friction.
2. Remove all covering from injured parts. Do not rub or break blisters.
3. Apply dressing to blisters.
4. Keep the injured area dry, protected, and elevated during transport. Do not allow coverings to come in direct contact with area.
5. Place gauze between fingers and toes.
6. Keep patient warm but not overheated.
7. Request paramedic evaluation if condition indicates (see Appendix 12).

HYPOTHERMIA

1. Check carotid pulse for at least 5 sec to determine pulselessness.
   a. If pulseless, initiate CPR.
   b. If pulse present, avoid CPR until pulse is lost.
2. Prevent further heat loss; remove from cold environment and move to warm area; cut off wet clothing and wrap in blankets, including head.
3. Administer high flow (10 to 15 LPM) of oxygen by mask resuscitation with mouth-to-pocket-mask; supplemental oxygen is preferred over bag-valve mask since this supplies warm air.
4. Paramedic evaluation required or transport immediately if paramedics unavailable.
5. Apply ECG monitor.
6. Handle patient gently. Rough movement can cause ventricular fibrillation.

SPECIAL CONSIDERATIONS

Frostbite

1. Partial rewarming is worse than none. Rarely should rewarming take place in the field.
2. Rewarming should be done under controlled conditions. It is extremely painful.

Hypothermia

1. No victim of hypothermia is considered dead until after rewarming.
2. When possible, all treatment should be left for a hospital setting.
3. If debrillation certified, and monitoring has been initiated, avoid CPR if an organized rhythm is identified even with the absence of a pulse.
4. CPR in severely hypothermic patients who have a pulse or electrical activity is likely to induce irreversible ventricular fibrillation.

Drowning and Near-Drowning

DESCRIPTION

Drowning is defined as death that occurs as a result of being in or under water. Near-drowning is submersion under water that does not result in death, and is the principal problem in all water-related accidents. All near-drowning victims will suffer from some degree of hypoxia or lack of oxygen. Common emergencies associated with near drowning are airway obstruction, cardiac arrest, heart attacks, head and neck injuries, internal injuries, and hypothermia.

SIGNIFICANT PHYSICAL FINDINGS

1. Alterations in level of consciousness, unconsciousness
2. Convulsions
3. Absent or abnormal respirations and pulse
4. Rales or signs of respiratory distress

5. Frothy pink sputum
6. Cough

SIGNIFICANT HISTORY

1. Length of submersion
2. Temperature of the water
3. Fresh or salt water
4. Specific aspects of incident (e.g., diving into shallow water)
5. Presence of drugs or alcohol

PATIENT CARE

1. If unconscious, suspect neck injury and treat appropriately.
   a. Establish an airway and initiate ventilations.
   b. Avoid hyperextension of the neck.
   c. Slide backboard under patient.
   d. Apply rigid cervical collar.
   e. Remove patient from water.
   f. Initiate CPR.
2. Expect vomiting, have suction available.
3. Administer high flow (10 to 15 LPM) of oxygen by mask.
4. Apply ECG monitor if EMT-D certified.
5. Consider an IV KVO.
6. Remove wet clothing
7. Paramedic evaluation required or transport immediately if paramedics unavailable.

SPECIAL CONSIDERATIONS

1. Initial resuscitation of the submersion victim is the same whether the near drowning occurred in salt water or in fresh water.
2. Alcohol intoxication is a major factor in adult drownings.
3. All near-drowning victims must be transported even if they appear fine. Delayed deaths due to pulmonary edema and aspiration pneumonia are not uncommon.
4. Proper stabilization and removal of the patient from the water is critical to preventing or avoiding further spinal injury.

Heat-Related Injuries

DESCRIPTION

Emergencies associated with excess heat (hyperthermia) result from the body's inability to cool itself normally by increasing respirations, surface blood flow, or perspiration. The most common emergencies associated with hyperthermia are heat syncope, heat cramps, heat exhaustion, and heat stroke.

1. *Heat syncope* or fainting results from vasodilitation and pooling of the blood in the lower extremities. Once the patient becomes horizontal, consciousness is regained and the patient recovers unless injured while falling. Treatment involves moving the patient to a cooler location.
2. *Heat cramps* result from the excessive loss of salt through perspiration. Muscular cramps can be mild to severe, involving the extremities or abdomen.
3. *Heat exhaustion* is significantly more serious, resulting in shock and possible coma. Pooling of blood in the skin and loss of water and salt through perspiration diminishes blood flow to vital organs, leading to hypovolemia.
4. *Heat stroke* is a life-threatening emergency brought about when the body's heat-regulating mechanisms fail to cool the body sufficiently.

SIGNIFICANT PHYSICAL FINDINGS

Heat Cramps

1. Weakness
2. Dizziness, faintness
3. Severe muscular cramps and pain

Heat Exhaustion

1. Rapid, shallow breathing
2. Rapid, weak pulse
3. Cold, clammy skin
4. Heavy perspiration
5. Total body weakness
6. Dizziness leading to unconsciousness

Heat Stroke

1. Confusion, disorientation, progressing to unconsciousness
2. Skin is usually hot and dry
3. Rapid, deep respirations
4. Rapid, weak pulse
5. Dilated pupils
6. Seizures

SIGNIFICANT HISTORY

1. Was collapse sudden or did symptoms develop gradually?
2. Surrounding circumstances: playing golf, jogging, prolonged exposure or exertion
3. Environmental conditions
4. Age of patient (elderly more susceptible to heat injuries)

PATIENT CARE

Heat Cramps

1. Move to a cooler area.
2. Instruct the patient to rest and lie down.
3. Contact base hospital to report findings and receive specific instructions.
4. Advise patient to increase intake of fluids if nausea is absent.

Heat Exhaustion/Heat Stroke

1. Move patient to a cooler area.
2. Remove enough clothing to cool patient.
3. Give patient salted water to drink only if conscious, alert, and not nauseated.
4. Position patient flat with legs elevated.
5. Treat for shock, but do not cover to point of overheating.
6. Request immediate paramedic evaluation if mental status deteriorates or patient unconscious and treat for heat stroke.

Heat Stroke

1. Cool rapidly in any manner with cold, wet sheets or ice packs.
2. Administer moderate flow (5 to 9 LPM) of oxygen by cannula or face mask.
3. Be prepared for possible seizures.
4. Apply ECG monitor if EMT-D authorized.
5. Consider an IV of normal saline.
6. Paramedic evaluation required or transport immediately if paramedics unavailable.

SPECIAL CONSIDERATIONS

1. Heat stroke is a true medical emergency and carries a high mortality rate.
2. Be aware that heat exhaustion can progress to heat stroke. Any change in mental status implies that the patient is suffering from heat stroke and must be cooled immediately.
3. Wet sheets over patient without good airflow will tend to increase patient's temperature.
4. Do not let cooling in the field delay transporting.

Inhalation Injuries

DESCRIPTION

Inhalation injuries can result from exposure to smoke, fire, or toxic gases. These injuries can lead to such life-threatening emergencies as upper airway obstruction, bronchospasm, pulmonary edema, carbon monoxide poisoning, shock, and respiratory or cardiac arrest. Victims of inhalation injuries, particularly from smoke, are at great risk for developing serious complications as late as 5 to 8 hours after the exposure.

SIGNIFICANT PHYSICAL FINDINGS

1. Skin or eye irritation
2. Shortness of breath, wheezing
3. Chest pain
4. Cough, black or "sooty"-looking sputum

5. Facial burns, burns of oral mucosa
6. Singed facial or nasal hairs
7. Hoarseness
8. Difficulty swallowing
9. Distinctive smoky or chemical breath odor
10. Chest tightness
11. Cherry red lips and mucosa indicative of carbon monoxide poisoning
12. Headache, confusion, irritability
13. Signs of shock: altered consciousness; rapid, weak pulse; cool, clammy skin; low blood pressure
14. Seizures
15. Nausea, vomiting

SIGNIFICANT HISTORY

1. Source of exposure
2. Exposed in a confined or enclosed space
3. Distinctive odor
4. Evidence of fire or smoke
5. Poor ventilation present
6. Length of time exposed

PATIENT CARE

1. Wear protective clothing and breathing apparatus if appropriate.
2. Remove patient from the scene.
3. Administer high flow (10 to 15 LPM) of oxygen by mask. Assist respirations as needed, particularly those with decreasing level of consciousness.
4. Protect and maintain airway.
5. Brush away all dry chemicals.
6. Remove contaminated clothing.
7. Irrigate and flush contaminated areas with lots of water.
8. Apply ECG monitor if EMT-D authorized.

9. Consider IV KVO.
10. Secure on a long backboard if patient unconscious and position on its side if necessary for airway maintenance.
11. Request paramedic evaluation if condition indicates (see Appendix 12).

SPECIAL CONSIDERATIONS

1. Carbon monoxide poisoning is the major cause of burn deaths that occur at the scene. Any unconscious burn victim should be assumed to be suffering from carbon monoxide poisoning requiring administration of high flow of oxygen.
2. All inhalation injuries must be medically evaluated since the body's reaction to smoke, fires, or toxic gases can be delayed for several hours.
3. Dry chemicals can react with water to form dangerous liquids; therefore, brush away all dry substances before flushing with copious amounts of water.
4. In the presence of toxic gases, evacuate everyone before treating any individual patient.

Mountain Sickness (High-Altitude Pulmonary Edema)

DESCRIPTION

This condition is found when respiratory distress begins due to a gain in altitude without the body having time to compensate for the difference. This is a treatable disease that can strike previously healthy skiers, climbers, and trekkers. Left untreated, it can be fatal.

SIGNIFICANT PHYSICAL FINDINGS

1. *Early signs:* fatigue, dyspnea at rest, dry cough, difficulty sleeping, loss of appetite, and headache; tachycardia at rest (pulse above 100)
2. *Late signs:* shortness of breath, cough with frothy pink sputum, dizziness, mental confusion, staggering gait, and coma

> **PATIENT CARE**
>
> 1. Give the patient supplemental oxygen.
> 2. Get the patient to a lower altitude. (As little as 1000 meters can make a great deal of difference.)

Scuba Diving Accidents

DESCRIPTION

Scuba diving (self-contained underwater breathing apparatus) is becoming a popular recreational sport for many people. As a result, more and more accidents are being treated each year. The most common medical emergencies associated with underwater diving are barotrauma, air embolism, pneumothorax, and decompression sickness (bends). These problems can occur any time that compressed air is used. The EMT must consider these possibilities any time a changing level of consciousness occurs in association with the use of compressed air.

1. *Barotrauma* is injury to the tissues of the air cavities with damage to the eardrum or sinuses resulting from excessive internal pressure during the descent.
2. *Air embolism* occurs when quick ascent causes pressure in the lungs to increase rapidly, rupturing alveoli and sending air bubbles throughout the circulatory system, blocking the flow of blood.
3. *Pneumothorax* can also result from rupturing alveoli.
4. *Decompression sickness (bends)* results from rapid ascent from depths greater than 30 feet and the formation of nitrogen bubbles, blocking circulation, especially involving the muscles and joints.

SIGNIFICANT PHYSICAL FINDINGS

Barotrauma

1. Mild to severe pain of affected area
2. A bloody or fluid discharge from the nose or ears

3. Dizziness
4. Hemorrhage from the tiny blood vessels in the eyes

Air Embolism/Pneumothorax

1. Blotching or itching of the skin
2. Frothy blood in the nose and mouth
3. Pain in the muscles, joints, and tendons; pain in the chest or abdomen
4. Dizziness
5. Vomiting
6. Blurred or distorted vision
7. Possible paralysis or coma
8. Difficulty breathing
9. Bloody sputum
10. Decreased breath sounds unilaterally
11. Air under skin of chest or neck
12. Diaphoresis

Decompression

1. Mottled skin
2. Rash
3. Headache
4. Severe pain in the joints and muscles, chest, and abdomen
5. Muscular cramps
6. Paralysis and/or numbness, indicating infarction of spinal cord
7. Unusually tired following a dive

SIGNIFICANT HISTORY

1. Depth of dive; number of dives in one day; length of time underwater
2. Previous problems encountered while diving
3. Significant medical history; history of asthma involves a higher incidence of air embolism due to air trapping
4. Current medications

PATIENT CARE

Barotrauma

1. Keep patient calm and quiet.
2. Position comfortably with head up.
3. Request paramedic evaluation if condition indicates (see Appendix 12).

Air Embolism/Pneumothorax

1. Provide basic life support as required.
2. Position patient on left side with head and chest lower than feet (prevents air from moving to lungs, heart, brain) if patient conscious.
3. Administer high flow (10 to 15 LPM) of oxygen by mask.
4. *Apply ECG monitor if EMT-D authorized.*
5. *Consider an IV D_5W KVO.*
6. Paramedic evaluation required; if parametics unavailable, transport immediately.

Compression

1. Provide basic life support as required.
2. Position on left side with chest and head lower than feet.
3. Administer high flow (10 to 15 LPM) of oxygen by mask.
4. *Apply ECG monitor if EMT-D authorized.*
5. *Consider an IV D_5W KVO.*
6. Paramedic evaluation required; if paramedics unavailable, transport immediately.

SPECIAL CONSIDERATIONS

1. Air embolism and decompression sickness require recompression in a hyperbaric chamber available. Notify the base hospital of possible condition so that arrangements can be made to transport patient to a facility with a hyperbaric chamber.
2. Any time that CPR is required with an emergency involving the use of compressed air, it is recommended that CPR be

performed in the Trendelenberg position—with head down and legs elevated approximately 30° or 12 inches.
3. Symptoms of an air embolism are usually apparent immediately upon surfacing, whereas symptoms of decompression illness take minutes to hours to become apparent.

MEDICAL EMERGENCIES

Abdominal Pain

DESCRIPTION

Abdominal pain can originate from problems associated with the cardiovascular system, gastrointestinal system, or genitourinary system. It can occur gradually or acutely. An "acute abdomen" refers to sudden and severe abdominal pain resulting from inflammation and irritation of the abdominal lining caused by the release of blood, acids, or feces from diseased or damaged organs. Causes of acute abdominal pain can include:

1. Aneurysm
2. Appendicitis
3. Ectopic pregnancy
4. Myocardial infarction
5. Ulcers
6. Ovarian cysts
7. Kidney stones

SIGNIFICANT PHYSICAL FINDINGS

1. Sick-looking patient, often in guarded or fetal position
2. Distended, rigid, or tender abdomen
3. Pulsating abdominal masses
4. Unequal or absent femoral pulses
5. Signs of shock: cool, clammy skin; rapid, weak pulse; altered consciousness; low blood pressure; paleness
6. Postural changes: pulse rise above 20 beats per minute, or a drop in systolic blood pressure greater than 20mmHg

7. Diaphoresis
8. Emesis

SIGNIFICANT HISTORY

1. Description of pain: severity, location, duration, radiation
2. Associated symptoms: nausea, vomiting of blood or "coffee ground" material; black, tarry, or bloody stools; diarrhea; constipation
3. Medical history: known ulcers, surgery, previous trauma, pregnancies, missed periods, hypertension, blood vessel disease, cardiac disease
4. Medications and allergies

PATIENT CARE

1. Position comfortably, generally on either side with knees drawn up.
2. Administer low flow (2 to 4 LPM) of oxygen by cannula.
3. Apply ECG monitor if EMT-D authorized.
4. Permit nothing by mouth.
5. Handle gently.
6. Take postural vital signs.
7. Treat for shock. If SBP below 90 and pulse rate above 110 or SBP below 80 regardless of pulse, apply and inflate antishock trousers if available.
8. Consider an IV.
9. Request paramedic evaluation if indicated by significant physical findings as listed in Appendix 12.

SPECIAL CONSIDERATIONS

1. Abdominal pain may be the first sign of impending rupture of an aneurysm, liver, spleen, or ectopic pregnancy and life-threatening hemorrhage. Monitor for signs of hypovolemic shock. Take postural vital signs.
2. Pulsating masses; gently palpate abdomen if aneurysm suspected.
3. Regardless of presenting vital signs, if aneurysm is suspected, immediate paramedic evaluation is required.

Alcohol-Related Emergencies

DESCRIPTION

Acute alcohol intoxication and alcohol withdrawal are the most serious emergencies associated with alcoholism. The main causes of death are aspiration of vomitus and respiratory depression. Alcohol intoxication is a result of an excess of alcohol in the blood. Alcohol withdrawal occurs when the patient cannot obtain alcohol, is too sick to drink, or abruptly stops drinking, resulting in a severe reaction ranging from delirium tremens (DTs) to seizures.

SIGNIFICANT PHYSICAL FINDINGS

ACUTE INTOXICATION

1. Odor of alcohol on patient's breath or clothing
2. Swaying and unsteady movement
3. Slurred speech, inability to carry on a conversation
4. Inappropriate or exaggerated behavior from giddiness to aggression and combativeness
5. Flushed appearance of the face; patient profusely sweating, complaining of feeling warm
6. Drowsiness
7. Nausea, vomiting
8. Danger signs indicating extreme emergency:
   a. Unconsciousness
   b. Breathing difficulties
   c. Fever
   d. Abnormal pulse rate, irregular pulse
   e. Vomiting while not fully conscious
   f. Convulsions

ACUTE WITHDRAWAL

1. Restlessness, disorientation, delusions
2. Tremors of the hands
3. Profuse sweating
4. Hallucinations
5. Convulsions
6. Hypotension

SIGNIFICANT HISTORY

1. History of alcoholism
2. Last drink taken and amount ingested:
   a. Withdrawal seizures can occur 5 to 48 hours after last drink.
   b. DTs occur as early as 2 to 4 days or as late as 7 to 10 days from last drink.
3. Medical history: diabetes, epilepsy, kidney disease, heart problems, ulcers
4. Current medications; any medications taken with alcohol? Are they taking Antabuse?
5. Medical alert tag

PATIENT CARE

ACUTE INTOXICATION

1. Protect patient from injury. Avoid restraints if possible. Request assistance from police if necessary. Stay alert to violent behavior.
2. Ensure an open airway and adequate respirations if patient unconscious. Watch for respiratory arrest.
3. Administer low flow (2 to 4 LPM) of oxygen by cannula.
4. Look for other injuries or medical problems.
5. Monitor vital signs and neurological status.
6. Secure patient to long backboard if unconscious, and position on its side if necessary for airway maintenance.

ACUTE WITHDRAWAL

1. Protect from injury if possible.
2. Avoid restraints if possible.
3. Ensure airway and assist respirations as needed.
4. Treat for shock. If SBP below 90 and pulse above 110, or SBP below 80 regardless of pulse, apply and inflate antishock trousers if available.
5. Treat seizures per protocols. If in status seizures, administer respirations and request paramedic evaluation.
6. Reinforce reality and tell the patient what you are doing. See if the patient is seeing things.

ACUTE INTOXICATION	ACUTE WITHDRAWAL
7. Protect airway from vomitus; have suction available.	7. Delirium tremens is a medical emergency. Paramedic evaluation required or transport immediately if paramedics unavailable.
8. Request paramedic evaluation if indicated by significant physical findings as listed in Appendix 12.	

SPECIAL CONSIDERATIONS

1. Some signs of alcohol abuse are similar to those found in medical emergencies. For instance, the "acetone" breath characteristic of diabetic coma can be mistaken for alcohol. Alcohol can always mask other medical problems.
2. Alcoholics commonly mix alcohol and drugs.
3. Do not leave an intoxicated patient unattended.
4. Assume that all threats of suicide or homicide are serious.
5. A calm, respectful attitude will reassure the patient that you are in control.
6. Do not engage in any argument with the patient.

ANEURYSMS (THORACIC AND ABDOMINAL)

DESCRIPTION

An aneurysm is a weakened section of the wall of an artery that becomes stretched with blood eventually tearing through the layers of the arterial wall (dissecting) or rupturing. Dissection refers to the passage of blood through a tear in the arterial wall, usually of the aorta between the inner and outer linings. Rupture of an aneurysm can lead to rapid, life-threatening internal bleeding as with an abdominal or thoracic aneurysm.

SIGNIFICANT PHYSICAL FINDINGS

THORACIC

1. Unequal or absent carotid, radial, or femoral pulses
2. Neurological signs suggesting a stroke
3. *Signs of shock:* rapid, weak pulse; altered consciousness; cool, clammy skin; low blood pressure; paleness
4. Distended neck veins, cyanosis of the neck and face
5. Differing blood pressures in each arm
6. Sudden onset of chest pain described as "tearing" or "through and through"

ABDOMINAL

1. Pulsating abdominal mass
2. Distended, rigid abdomen
3. *Signs of shock:* rapid, weak pulse; altered consciousness; cool, clammy skin; low blood pressure; paleness
4. Diminished, unequal, or absent pulses in the lower extremities
5. Sudden onset of acute and severe abdominal pain

SIGNIFICANT HISTORY

THORACIC

1. History of hypertension
2. Severe pain beginning in the chest and progressing toward the legs or into the back
3. Sudden onset of back pain in older patients

ABDOMINAL

1. History of arteriosclerotic disease or abdominal aneurysm
2. Severe abdominal pain radiating to the lower back

PATIENT CARE

1. Administer high flow (10 to 15 LPM) of oxygen by mask. Assist respirations as needed.
2. Treat for shock. If SBP below 90 and pulse above 110 or SBP below 80 regardless of pulse, apply and inflate anti-shock trousers if available.

3. Consider starting an IV with large-bore needle.
4. Apply ECG monitor if EMT-D authorized.
5. Avoid deep abdominal palpation.
6. Handle gently.
7. Obtain blood pressure on both arms for baseline. Check femoral pulses for presence and equalness.
8. Paramedic evaluation required; if paramedics unavailable, transport immediately.

SPECIAL CONSIDERATIONS

1. Cardiac tamponade can be a complication of a dissecting thoracic aneurysm requiring immediate paramedic intervention or transport. Signs and symptoms of tamponade are:
   a. Severe cyanosis above the nipple line
   b. Distended neck veins
   c. Distant heart sounds
   d. Narrowing pulse pressure (systolic and diastolic pressure move closer together)
2. Because of intense and severe pain, treating the patient will be difficult. Unless in shock or respiratory distress, allow the patient to assume position of comfort.

Behavioral Emergencies

DESCRIPTION

A behavioral emergency exists when a patient displays unusual, bizarre, or inappropriate behavior that is dangerous to others or self or overwhelms the individual's ability to deal rationally with the immediate situation. Alcohol intoxication, drug use, and certain medical illnesses can mimic or worsen existing personality disorders or trigger threatening behavior. Depression, suicide, aggression, violence, and acute anxiety are the most common emergencies encountered in the field. In addition, victims of crime may also present with an overwhelming emotional emergency requiring immediate intervention and support.

SIGNIFICANT PHYSICAL FINDINGS

1. Withdrawn, not responding to people or environment
2. Hostile or aggressive: tries to hurt self or others

3. Anxious and fearful
   a. Profuse sweating
   b. Flushed appearance
   c. Rapid pulse and respirations
   d. Hyperventilation
   e. Rapid speech
4. Hallucinating (seeing things that are not there or hearing voices that are not real)
5. Crying or hysterical

SIGNIFICANT HISTORY

1. History of recent crisis, emotional trauma, illness, changes in behavior, suicidal ideas
2. Alcohol or drug use
3. Exposure to toxic substances
4. Previous psychiatric disorders, medical problems, medication
5. Family history of psychiatric disorders
6. Current physician or psychiatrist

PATIENT CARE

1. Ensure everyone's safety. Request assistance from local law enforcement agency if necessary.
2. Stay calm and evaluate the situation.
3. Identify yourself. Speak slowly and clearly.
4. Treat life-threatening emergencies.
5. Eliminate the possibility of other illnesses or injuries that might account for behavior [i.e., hypoxia (lack of oxygen), hypoglycemia (insulin shock), head injury, stroke].
6. Foster effective communication.
   a. Express your desire to help. Speak in brief, clear sentences.
   b. Maintain eye contact.
   c. Listen to what the patient is saying.
   d. Give calm, relaxed reassurance.
   e. Never use physical force unless the patient is a threat to himself or others.
7. For suicidal patients:
   a. Stay with the patient at all times.
   b. Take the threat seriously; listen to the patient.

c. Remove all dangerous objects.
   d. Transport to the hospital.
8. For aggressive and violent patients:
   a. Request assistance from local law enforcement agency.
   b. Avoid approaching a potentially violent patient alone.
   c. Avoid aggressive actions unless there is the immediate possibility of serious injury.
   d. Restrain a patient only if there is adequate assistance to do so safely and according to local protocols (see Appendix 14).
   e. Maintain a neutral approach; avoid any action that might threaten the patient.
   f. Avoid placing any obstacles between the patient and the only doorway; feeling trapped may worsen the patient's hostility.
   g. Avoid turning your back; do not isolate yourself from other rescuers.
9. For patients needing treatment and transport but are uncooperative; request intervention from local law enforcement agency. Police must place patient under protective custody before treatment and transportation can be accomplished.
10. Explain the situation to the patient and what you plan to do.
11. Contact the base hospital for transporting instructions.
12. Transport to the appropriate facility.

SPECIAL CONSIDERATIONS

1. Not all hospitals are equipped to handle behavioral emergencies. Contact the base hospital prior to transport to determine the appropriate facility.
2. Keep voice calm and at a normal or low speaking volume. This helps reduce a patient's agitation and hold the patient's attention.

Coma

DESCRIPTION

Coma is the complete state of unconsciousness. In this state the patient loses the reflexes that protect the airway from aspiration and obstruction, requiring great care in establishing an airway and ensuring adequate breathing. The causes of coma are many: trauma, diabetes, stroke, meningitis, seizures, alcoholic intoxication, drug overdose, or other medical problems involving the thyroid, kidneys, or adrenal glands.

SIGNIFICANT PHYSICAL FINDINGS

1. Medical alert bracelet or necklace
2. Evidence of traumatic injury and mechanism of injury
3. Breath odor: fruity odor may indicate diabetes and hyperglycemia; alcoholic odor does not necessarily mean that the coma is a result of alcohol
4. Hypertension (BP above 160/90) or hypotension (SBP below 90)
5. Evidence of drug use: needle tracks, drug paraphernalia
6. Abnormal/unusual breathing pattern

SIGNIFICANT HISTORY

1. Report from relatives or bystanders as to unusual behavior prior to unconsciousness, changes in behavior or mood
2. History of hypertension, recent illness, fever
3. Drugs, liquor bottles, medications in the immediate environment

---

PATIENT CARE

1. Establish and maintain an airway using cervical spine precautions. Insert an oropharyngeal airway if gag reflex absent. Have suction available.
2. Immobilize neck and spine for all suspected trauma.
3. Administer moderate to high flow (5 to 15 LPM) of oxygen and assist respirations as needed.
4. Apply ECG monitor.
5. Immobilize on long backboard and position on its side if necessary for airway maintenance.
6. Consider an IV.
7. Paramedic evaluation required; if paramedics unavailable, transport immediately.

Diabetic Emergencies

DESCRIPTION

Diabetes mellitus is a condition caused by decreased insulin production. This condition cannot be cured, only controlled through diet or insulin injections. The diabetic taking insulin is at great risk for developing diabetic coma or insulin shock. Both problems can be life threatening.

Diabetic coma results from a decreased insulin supply and an excessively high blood sugar level (hyperglycemia). Adequate insulin is not being produced by the body, or the person is not taking enough insulin.

Insulin shock occurs when there is too much insulin in the blood, or a seriously low blood sugar level (hypoglycemia). This can happen if the diabetic does not eat enough, takes too much insulin, is ill or has a fever, or overexercises.

SIGNIFICANT PHYSICAL FINDINGS

DIABETIC COMA (HYPERGLYCEMIA)	INSULIN SHOCK (HYPOGLYCEMIA)
1. Signs of air hunger: rapid deep breaths with frequent sighing	1. Headache, dizziness
2. Sweet or fruity odor on breath, like nail polish remover	2. Normal or shallow breathing
3. Rapid, weak pulse	3. Normal blood pressure
4. Normal or slightly low blood pressure	4. Normal or rapid pulse
5. Dehydration, dry mouth	5. Hostility, aggression, apathy, unconsciousness
6. Red, dry, warm skin	6. Extreme weakness
7. Vomiting	7. Pale, moist skin
8. Abdominal pain	8. Excessive salivation or drooling
9. Confusion, disorientation, restlessness	9. Fainting
10. Intense thirst, frequent urination	10. Tingling and numbness in fingers or feet
11. Dim vision	11. Double vision
12. Coma	12. Absence of thirst

SIGNIFICANT HISTORY

1. Confirm history of diabetes; if unconscious, look for med-tags
2. If taking insulin, time and amount of last dose; usual amount taken; oral hypoglycemics
3. Recent illnesses, hospitalizations, surgeries, injuries
4. Past problems associated with diabetes
5. Onset of present illness: sudden or gradual

PATIENT CARE

DIABETIC COMA (HYPERGLYCEMIA)	INSULIN SHOCK (HYPOGLYCEMIA)
1. Establish and maintain airway. Administer moderate flow (5 to 9 LPM) of oxygen by cannula or mask.	1. If patient is conscious, give any form of sugar (i.e., orange juice, soft drinks with sugar, candy, sugar cubes, or plain sugar).
2. Have suction available. Be alert for vomiting.	2. If patient is unconscious, establish an airway and assist respirations.
3. Treat for complications such as shock and seizures.	3. Have suction available. Be alert for vomiting.
4. Apply ECG monitor.	4. Apply ECG monitor.
5. Consider starting an IV.	5. Consider starting an IV.
6. Paramedic evaluation required or transport immediately if paramedics unavailable.	6. Paramedic evaluation required; if paramedics unavailable, transport immediately.

SPECIAL CONSIDERATIONS

1. The diabetic will frequently know what is needed. *Listen to the patient.*
2. Insulin shock is more critical than diabetic coma. The onset of diabetic coma is over several days, whereas the onset of insulin shock is sudden. The patient in insulin shock desperately needs intravenous glucose before brain damage and

death occur. It is often difficult to decide the exact condition of the diabetic patient without a blood sugar test. Do not waste time deciding which condition exists. If in doubt, treat the patient for insulin shock, and get them to a hospital.

3. For patients who are unconscious, avoid any oral sugar agent due to possible aspiration or airway obstruction.

Drug Abuse and Overdose

DESCRIPTION

Drug abuse is the self-administration of drugs for purposes other than medical use. Overdose is an excess of a drug taken which has harmful effects. An overdose can be accidental or intentional. Often, drugs are taken in combination or with alcohol. Drug withdrawal is a serious problem of habitual drug abuse.

Categories of commonly abused drugs are as follows:

Uppers (stimulants): amphetamines, decongestants, antidepressants, ritalin, caffeine, cocaine

Downers (depressants): qualude, barbituates, alcohol, antihistamines, tranquilizers

Narcotics (pain relievers): heroine, percodan, talwin, demerol, methadone, pain cocktails

Hallucinogens (mind-altering): LSD, marijuana, PCP, "designer" drugs, mushrooms

Volatile chemicals (sniffed or inhaled): airplane glue, cleaning fluids, solvents

Most of the time, the EMT will be unable to tell exactly which drug a patient has been using. Do not delay treatment while trying to identify a drug; treat the patient first. Look for clues in the patient's environment. Seek information from others. Remember that symptoms of drug and alcohol abuse mimic those of other medical emergencies. Guidelines for treatment generally apply to both alcohol and drug abuse.

SIGNIFICANT PHYSICAL FINDINGS

Signs and symptoms of drug overdose vary depending on the drug taken.

DRUG OVERDOSE	DRUG WITHDRAWAL

1. *Uppers:* Excitement, increased pulse and respiratory rates, rapid speech, dry mouth, dilated pupils, sweating, lack of sleep, seizures; cocaine use can cause nasal congestion
2. *Downers:* sluggishness, sleepiness, lacking coordination of body and speech, slow pulse and respirations, respiratory depression or arrest
3. *Hallucinogens:* fast pulse, dilated pupils, flushed face, nonsensical conversation, patient "sees" things, little concept of real time, aggressive or fearful
4. *Narcotics:* slowed pulse and respirations, lowered skin temperature, constricted pupils, relaxed muscles, profuse sweating, sleepiness
5. *Volatile chemicals:* dazed or showing temporary loss of contact with reality, swollen membranes or possible coma, patient complains of numb mouth and feeling or tingling inside head, arrhythmias, runny nose

1. Shaking
2. Anxiety
3. Nausea
4. Confusion, irritability
5. Profuse sweating
6. Increased pulse and respiratory rates

SIGNIFICANT HISTORY

1. If patient unconscious, question bystanders about what was seen.

2. Was alcohol involved?
3. What was taken, how much, and by what route?
4. Has this happened before?
5. Did the patient vomit already?
6. Did the patient have a seizure?
7. Other medical problems
8. Current medications, allergies
9. Currently under psychiatric care

PATIENT CARE

1. Treatment for drug abuse and overdose is the same regardless of drug taken.
2. Talk with patient to gain his confidence and help maintain his level of consciousness.
3. Ensure open airway and adequate respirations. Monitor closely for respiratory depression and arrest.
4. Administer high flow (10 to 15 LPM) of oxygen by mask.
5. Call the base hospital of your provider group for specific instructions.
6. Anticipate vomiting; have suction available. Take great care to prevent aspiration.
7. Apply ECG monitor.
8. Consider an IV of normal saline or lactated Ringer's solution.
9. Treat for shock. If SBP below 90 and pulse above 110, or SBP below 80 regardless of pulse, apply and inflate antishock trousers if available.
10. Monitor vital signs closely and level of consciousness. Watch for seizures.
11. Protect the patient from hurting himself or others.
12. Observe patient at all times. Never leave an intoxicated patient alone.
13. Move patient to quiet area if agitated.
14. Explain each step of care to help reduce the paranoia of the patient.
15. Search the area for items that might be useful in identifying drugs taken.
16. Request paramedic evaluation if indicated by significant physical findings as listed in Appendix 12.

SPECIAL CONSIDERATIONS

1. Many drug abusers may appear calm at first and then become violent as time passes. Be alert and ready to protect yourself.
2. Be particularly cautious and alert when dealing with PCP or phencyclidine (angel dust, killer weed, horse tranquilizer). Users who are prone to aggressive and violent acts should be kept in a quiet, nonstimulating environment. Do not try to "talk down" these patients since this tends to aggravate them further.
3. Attempt to identify drug taken but do not delay treatment.
4. If ipecac is required, see Appendix 18.

Hypertensive Emergencies

DESCRIPTION

A hypertensive emergency is the sudden elevation of a person's blood pressure—a systolic BP above 180 and a diastolic BP above 120—with accompanying signs and symptoms. Stress or disease can increase the blood pressure so much that rupture or damage to the arteries, particularly in the brain, will occur. If untreated, a hypertensive emergency can lead to convulsions, coma, and death.

SIGNIFICANT PHYSICAL FINDINGS

1. Elevated blood pressure
2. Pregnancy
3. Signs and symptoms of pulmonary edema:
   a. Frothy pink sputum
   b. Rales/noisy respirations
   c. Dyspnea
   d. Rapid respiratory rate
4. Headache, blurred vision
5. Confusion, anxiety
6. Evidence of head trauma
7. Chest pain
8. Abdominal pain or back pain
9. Nausea, vomiting
10. Signs and symptoms of a stroke:
    a. Paralysis

b. Numbness
   c. Impaired speech
   d. Altered behavior
   e. Unsteady walk, clumsiness
11. Altered level of consciousness
12. Seizures

SIGNIFICANT HISTORY

1. Known history of hypertension; what is different this time
2. Abrupt cessation of antihypertensive medications
3. First pregnancies or problems with previous pregnancies
4. Medical history: angina, heart disease, kidney disease, hyperthyroidism, aneurysms
5. Current medications

PATIENT CARE

1. Maintain airway and adequate respirations.
2. Administer high flow (10 to 15 LPM) of oxygen unless history of COPD.
3. Apply ECG monitor.
4. Consider an IV of D_5W at KVO.
5. Monitor and record vital signs with neurological checks frequently. Take a series of BP measurements.
6. Minimize stimulation and noise. Keep patient calm. Darken patient area if possible.
7. Position comfortably with head elevated or on one side.
8. Anticipate and treat appropriately for seizures.
9. Have suction available for vomiting.
10. Paramedic evaluation required; if paramedics unavailable, transport immediately.

SPECIAL CONSIDERATIONS

1. Normal blood pressure measurements:
   a. *Healthy adult male:* SBP 120 to 150 mmHg, DBP 65 to 90 mmHg.

    b. *Healthy adult female:* SBP 110 to 140 mmHg, DBP 55 to 80 mmHg.
    c. *Rough estimate:* Add 100 to the age of the patient for SBP.
2. Hypertension is found in over one-half of all stroke patients.
3. Hypertension is often associated with stroke, aortic aneurysm, congestive heart failure, and angina.
4. Hypertensive emergencies can exist with blood pressures less than 180/120. Look for the presence of other symptoms.

Seizures

DESCRIPTION

A seizure or convulsion is the sudden onset of involuntary muscle activity, ranging from diffuse and violent muscular contraction (tonic) and relaxation (clonic) to localized muscular twitching and jerking. The more generalized tonic–clonic seizures are followed by postictal unconsciousness and then confusion as is characteristic of a grand mal seizure. Status seizure is continuous prolonged seizure activity or recurrent generalized seizures in which the individual never fully returns to an alert state between each seizure.

SIGNIFICANT PHYSICAL FINDINGS

1. Ongoing seizure activity, or seizure lasting longer than 5 minutes
2. Incontinence
3. Unconsciousness, disorientation, confusion
4. Head and mouth trauma
5. Pregnancy
6. Medical alert tag

SIGNIFICANT HISTORY

1. *Seizure activity:* first seizure; how long it lasted; what the seizure was like; previous seizure history
2. *Medical history:* head trauma, diabetes, headaches, drugs and alcohol use, medications, pregnancies

PATIENT CARE

1. Protect the patient from injury. Remove hazardous objects. Lay patient on floor or ground. Do not restrain. Loosen restrictive clothing.
2. Ensure a patient airway and adequate respirations. Do not force anything in mouth or between teeth.
3. Administer moderate flow (5 to 9 LPM) or high flow (10 to 15 LPM) of oxygen if in status seizure.
4. Apply ECG monitor.
5. Consider starting an IV of lactated Ringer's or normal saline solution.
6. Contact private physician if patient under medical care for seizures.
7. Secure patient on backboard and position appropriately for airway maintenance.
8. Paramedic evaluation required or transport immediately if paramedics unavailable for the following:
    a. Status seizure
    b. Pregnant female
    c. First-time seizure
    d. Repetitive seizures

SPECIAL CONSIDERATIONS

1. Bite blocks are not recommended. Most patients do not bite their tongue during a seizure.
2. Seizures in a pregnant woman is a true emergency requiring paramedic evaluation or immediate transport.
3. Ask orienting questions as soon as possible: "What is your name, age, birth date; where are you; what is the day, month, and year?" Repeat the same questions as time passes to see how oriented the patient is becoming.
4. Usual recovery sequence:
    a. Patient becomes more alert but is disoriented as to person, place, and time.
    b. Patient starts remembering personal information first: name, age, birth date.
    c. Patient starts remembering more general information.

Stroke (CVA)

DESCRIPTION

A stroke, also known as a CVA or cerebrovascular accident, results when the blood supply to any portion of the brain is interrupted enough to cause damage. The most common causes of a stroke are: blood clots, hemorrhage from a ruptured or torn artery, and compression of brain tissue from brain tumors or trauma. The resulting disability will depend on the site and amount of brain damaged.

SIGNIFICANT PHYSICAL FINDINGS

1. Headache
2. Confusion, dizziness, coma
3. Loss of function of extremities on one or both sides
4. Collapse
5. Mouth drawn to one side of the face or drooping on one side; paralysis of facial muscles, resulting in loss of expression
6. Impaired speech
7. Impaired vision
8. Personality changes
9. Rapid, strong pulse
10. Difficult respirations
11. Pupils unequal in size or reaction
12. Face usually flushed or pale
13. Loss of bladder or bowel control
14. Nausea, vomiting
15. Hallucinations
16. Blood pressure measures different readings in each arm

SIGNIFICANT HISTORY

1. Presence of preliminary signs and symptoms as reported by patient: headache, weakness, clumsiness, sudden or unexplained dizziness, nausea
2. Changes in personality or moods as reported by family

3. Medical history: hypertension, heart disease, trauma
4. Current medications

PATIENT CARE

1. Ensure an open airway and adequate respirations.
2. Insert oral airway if patient unconscious and gag reflex is absent. Have suction available.
3. Administer high flow (10 to 15 LPM) of oxygen by mask.
4. Apply ECG monitor.
5. Position on back with head and shoulders slightly elevated (30° or 12 inches) if conscious; if unconscious, secure on a long backboard and position appropriately for airway maintenance.
6. Monitor vital signs, check both carotid pulses gently for equalness.
7. Give nothing by mouth; remove all dentures and false teeth.
8. Keep the patient warm but do not overheat.
9. Keep the patient absolutely quiet. Handle gently. Support paralyzed limbs when lifting and moving.
10. Avoid unnecessary movement.
11. Paramedic evaluation required if history of cardiac disease, respiratory distress, or unconsciousness.
12. Consider starting an IV of D_5W at KVO.

SPECIAL CONSIDERATIONS

1. *Note the patient's state of consciousness.* Massive strokes involving the brain stem will render a patient completely unconscious.
2. The conscious CVA patient may not be able to speak to you but probably can hear and understand what is going on around. Be supportive and communicative, but avoid saying anything that will worsen anxiety.
3. High blood pressure accompanied by a slow pulse is an indication of marked brain swelling. Paramedic evaluation or immediate transport is critical.

OBSTETRICAL EMERGENCIES

Emergency Normal Childbirth

DESCRIPTION

Delivering a baby in the field can be an emergency event for which there is little time to prepare and transport. If delivery can be expected within 5 minutes, the EMT should delay transporting and prepare to assist the mother.

SIGNIFICANT PHYSICAL FINDINGS AND HISTORY

Based on the following observations, determine whether delivery is imminent:

1. Rectal fullness or sensation of need to have a bowel movement
2. Contractions less than 2 minutes apart
3. Crowning or bulging of the fetal head or presentation of any part in the vagina
4. Rupture of amniotic sac or "bag of waters" (indicates final stage of labor, but does not necessarily signal imminent delivery)
5. Labor for first babies averages 12 to 17 hours

PATIENT CARE

Delivery of the Baby

If delivery imminent, within 5 to 15 minutes, request paramedics.

1. Position and drape the mother.
2. Open the OB kit; wash hands (if possible) before putting on gloves.
3. Drape sterile towels under buttocks, between legs, across abdomen, and over each thigh.
4. Have bulb syringe nearby to suction infant as head emerges.

5. At appearance of head, place the palm of your hand over the head of the baby and apply gentle pressure to prevent forceful delivery of the head. Avoid pressure against the fontanelles or soft spots.
6. If amniotic sac does not break, use clamp or finger to puncture and push sac away from baby's mouth.
7. Check umbilical cord; if wrapped around neck, gently loosen it and slip it over the head carefully. If it is too tight to be slipped over the head, the cord should be clamped at two sites 2 inches apart and cut between the clamps.
8. Once the head is visible, suction the baby's mouth and each nostril with the bulb syringe, inserting no more than $\frac{1}{2}$ inch into the nostrils and 1 to $1\frac{1}{2}$ inches in the mouth). Δ CTO suction mouth first, then nostrils. *Note:* Squeeze air from syringe before inserting into nose or mouth.
9. If shoulders prove difficult, slight traction on baby's head toward the floor should be applied for upper shoulder, and for the lower shoulder traction should be toward the ceiling.
10. The infant will be extremely slippery. Handle with caution, supporting the head with one hand, the abdomen and hips with the other hand. Keep head lower than trunk to facilitate drainage from mouth and nose.
11. Wipe face. Suction mouth and nose again.
12. If infant does not begin breathing at this point, stimulate it by rubbing its back or snapping the soles of its feet. If still no response, start mouth-to-mouth/nose ventilations using very small breaths.
13. Place the infant on its side between the mother's legs on a firm surface with its head slightly lower than its body.
14. If infant is breathing normally, clamp and cut the umbilical cord after pulsations cease. Place two clamps on the cord about 2 inches apart, positioned about 6 inches from the baby's navel. Cut with sterile scissors from OB kit.
15. Wrap infant in blanket and keep warm, letting the mother hold.
16. Check for presence of twins.
17. Place sterile pad between mother's legs.

Delivery of the Placenta

1. Do not delay transporting while awaiting delivery of placenta.
2. Do not pull on the cord to check separation of placenta.
3. When delivered, wrap in a plastic bag and transport with mother to hospital.

Care of the Newborn

1. Keep warm by drying infant and wrapping in warmed blankets (if possible), covering head as well. If in home, use clothes dryer to warm blankets.
2. Do not administer oxygen unless needed for ventilation or special circumstances.
3. Suction airway. Suction mouth first, then nostrils, using bulb syringe from OB kit, squeeze air from syringe before suctioning, and insert no more than $\frac{1}{2}$ inches into nostrils and suction. Repeat for mouth, inserting 1 to $1\frac{1}{2}$ inches.

Resuscitation of the Newborn

1. If no spontaneous respirations begin in 30 seconds after delivery, begin mouth-to-mouth/mouth-to-nose ventilations while keeping the baby covered as much as possible.
2. Apply CPR if no brachial pulse palpated.
3. Continue resuscitation until breathing starts; then apply 2 to 3 liters via nasal cannula or mask held just above face.

SPECIAL CONSIDERATIONS

1. Delivery of the placenta may take as long as 30 minutes. Begin transporting as soon as mother and child are stable.
2. If CPR becomes necessary for infant, one EMT should begin resuscitation while a second EMT clamps and cuts the cord.
3. The greatest risks to the newborn infant are *airway obstruction* and *hypothermia*. Keep baby covered, warm, and dry; keep airway suctioned with bulb syringe. Keep aid vehicle warm with heaters on, even in the summertime.
4. Greatest risk to mother is postpartum hemorrhage. Watch for signs of shock and excessive vaginal bleeding.

Prepartum Hemorrhage

DESCRIPTION

Prepartum hemorrhage means bleeding during pregnancy or immediately before the birth of the baby. The causes for early bleeding are ruptured uterus, abruptive placenta, or placenta previa.

SIGNIFICANT PHYSICAL FINDINGS

1. External vaginal bleeding
2. Abdominal rigidity
3. Relaxed uterus during a contraction
4. Falling blood pressure, hypotension
5. Signs of shock: cool, clammy skin; weak, fast pulse; altered consciousness; paleness

SIGNIFICANT HISTORY

1. Intermittent spotting or bleeding
2. Sudden onset of abdominal pain
3. History of previous cesarean section

PATIENT CARE

1. Administer high flow (10 to 15 LPM) of oxygen by mask.
2. Treat for shock. If SBP below 90 and pulse above 110, or SBP below 80 regardless of pulse, apply and inflate medical antishock trousers if available. Do not inflate abdominal section unless systolic blood pressure less than 80 mm HG.
3. Apply ECG monitor.
4. Position mother on either side with legs elevated if MAST not in use.
5. Consider an IV of S_5W KVO.
6. Monitor vital signs frequently.
7. Paramedic evaluation required; if paramedics unavailable, transport immediately.

SPECIAL CONSIDERATIONS

1. Even though external blood loss may be minimal, severe internal hemorrhage may result. Blood pressure and pulse are good indicators of condition.
2. Having the mother lay flat can worsen shock and severely interrupt blood flow to the fetus. Unless using MAST, position on either side.
3. This is a true emergency and must be treated aggressively by paramedics or emergency room personnel.

Breech Delivery

DESCRIPTION

A breech birth refers to a delivery in which the presenting part is the buttocks or limbs instead of the head.

SIGNIFICANT PHYSICAL FINDING

An arm, leg, or the buttocks appear in the vagina.

PATIENT CARE

Frank Breech—Buttocks First

1. Allow buttocks and trunk to deliver spontaneously.
2. Support the legs and trunk.
3. If head does not deliver in 3 minutes:
   a. Raise body toward ceiling until face protrudes; *NEVER attempt to pull baby from the vagina.*
   b. If head still does not deliver, create an air passage by inserting two fingers into the vagina, forming a "V" on either side of the infant's nose and pushing against the vagina, away from the baby's face.
4. Transport immediately with mother's buttocks elevated. *Do not remove hand until relieved by hospital staff.*

Limb Presentation
No attempt should be made to deliver in the field.

1. Place mother on either side with legs and buttocks elevated as much as tolerated.

2. Administer high flow (10 to 15 LPM) of oxygen by mask.
3. Paramedic assistance required; if paramedics unavailable, transport immediately.
4. Notify hospital enroute so they can prepare for cesarean.

SPECIAL CONSIDERATION

A breech delivery can be serious and become life threatening. Do not delay transporting if baby's head does not deliver in 3 minutes.

Prolapsed Cord

DESCRIPTION

Prolapsed cord refers to the situation in which the umbilical cord comes out of the birth canal before the baby. Emergency care is urgent since the baby is in danger of suffocation from pressure on the cord.

SIGNIFICANT PHYSICAL FINDINGS AND HISTORY

1. Amniotic sac has already broken
2. Umbilical cord visibly protruding from vagina

PATIENT CARE

1. Place mother in knee-chest position with buttocks in the air, or lying on either side with hips elevated.
2. Administer high flow (10 to 15 LPM) of oxygen to mother by mask.
3. Wrap a sterile towel (preferably moisten in sterile saline) around the visible portion of the cord.
4. If no pulsations felt in the cord, put on sterile glove and insert two fingers between the cord and vagina to relieve pressure.
5. Maintain pressure on baby's head (avoid exerting pressure on the fontanelles, or soft spots) until medics arrive or until relieved by the hospital staff.
6. Paramedic evaluation required; if paramedics unavailable, transport immediately.

Cord around the Neck

DESCRIPTION

The umbilical cord becomes wrapped around the baby's neck in the birth canal. The greatest concern is that the baby would be strangulated by the cord.

SIGNIFICANT PHYSICAL FINDING

As the infant's head emerges from the vagina, the cord is visibly wrapped around its neck.

PATIENT CARE

1. Attempt to slip the cord over the baby's head.
2. If the cord is too tight, clamp the cord at two sites 2 inches apart and cut between the clamps.
3. Unwrap the cord from around the neck.
4. Paramedic evaluation required; if paramedics unavailable, transport immediately.

Postpartum Hemorrhage

DESCRIPTION

Postpartum hemorrhage refers to excessive internal or external bleeding following the delivery of the infant.

SIGNIFICANT PHYSICAL FINDINGS

1. External bleeding from vagina in excess of five soaked pads within 30 minutes
2. Abdominal rigidity or tenderness, suggesting internal hemorrhage
3. Signs of shock: rapid, weak pulse; altered consciousness; cool, clammy skin; low blood pressure; paleness

SIGNIFICANT HISTORY

1. History of problems or bleeding anytime during pregnancy
2. Previous cesarean section

3. Severe pain anywhere
4. Intense thirst

PATIENT CARE

1. Massage lower abdomen firmly with a circular motion.
2. Treat for shock. If SBP below 90 and pulse above 110 or SBP below 80 regardless of pulse, apply and inflate anti-shock trousers if available.
3. Administer high flow (10 to 15 LPM) of oxygen by mask.
4. Place sanitary napkin at opening of vagina. Once in place, *do not remove,* but add additional pads as necessary.
5. Do not hold legs together or put anything into vagina.
6. Preserve any tissue passed.
7. Paramedic evaluation required; if paramedics unavailable, transport immediately.

SPECIAL CONSIDERATIONS

1. Even though external blood loss may be minimal, severe internal hemorrhage may result. Blood pressure and pulse are good indicators of condition. Look for signs of shock: altered consciousness; rapid, weak pulse; cool, clammy skin; low blood pressure; paleness.
2. This is a true emergency and must be treated by paramedics or emergency room personnel.

Premature Birth

DESCRIPTION

An infant weighing less than $5\frac{1}{2}$ pounds at birth, or any infant born before the seventh month of pregnancy, is considered to be premature. Premature babies are susceptible to respiratory disease and infections and therefore require special care.

SIGNIFICANT PHYSICAL FINDINGS AND HISTORY

1. Thinner, smaller, and redder than full term
2. Disproportionately large head to rest of body

PATIENT CARE

1. Keep infant warm.
2. Keep airway clear.
3. Administer oxygen at 2 to 3 LPM by placing nasal cannula or face mask close to infant's face.
4. Observe umbilical cord closely for signs of bleeding and apply additional clamps if needed.
5. Avoid contamination—wear sterile mask to prevent transmission of illnesses to infant.
6. Paramedic evaluation required; if paramedics unavailable, transport immediately.

SPECIAL CONSIDERATIONS

The greatest risks to the newborn infant are airway obstruction and hypothermia. Keep baby covered, warm, and dry; keep airway suctioned with bulb syringe.

Multiple Births

DESCRIPTION

Twins are not a complication if the deliveries proceed normally. More than two children may be associated with small size and complications.

SIGNIFICANT PHYSICAL FINDINGS AND HISTORY

1. Very large abdomen after one baby is delivered
2. Return of strong labor contractions within 10 minutes after the first baby is born

PATIENT CARE

1. Cut and clamp cord of first child and proceed with second delivery.
2. Keep infants warm.

3. Administer 2 to 3 LPM of oxygen via mask or nasal cannula held above head.
  4. Paramedic evaluation required; if paramedics unavailable, transport immediately.

Spontaneous Abortion

DESCRIPTION

Spontaneous abortion (also referred to as a miscarriage) is the loss of a pregnancy before the twenty-eighth week of gestation.

SIGNIFICANT PHYSICAL FINDINGS AND HISTORY

1. Heavy vaginal bleeding—in excess of three pads per hour
2. Passage of tissue
3. Cramplike pains in lower abdomen
4. Patient's knowledge of pregnancy
5. Signs of shock: altered consciousness; rapid weak pulse; cool, clammy skin; low blood pressure; paleness
6. Postural changes in vital signs (see Appendix 13)

PATIENT CARE

1. Administer high flow (10 to 15 LPM) of oxygen.
2. Place a sanitary napkin over vaginal opening. Do not pack the vagina.
3. Treat for shock.
4. If SBP below 90 and pulse above 110, or SBP below 80 regardless of pulse, apply and inflate antishock trousers, including abdominal section, if available.
5. Save any tissue passed and soaked pads.
6. Request paramedic evaluation if indicated by significant physical findings as listed in Appendix 12. These patients need to be medically evaluated.

SPECIAL CONSIDERATIONS

Loss of a pregnancy can be very traumatic and emotionally upsetting. Use discretion when referring to this loss as an abortion, as such terminology can be offensive and carries strong negative connotations.

Ectopic Pregnancy

DESCRIPTION

Ectopic pregnancy occurs when the fertilized egg implants somewhere outside the uterus (i.e., the abdominal cavity, the fallopian tube, or the ovary). Such a pregnancy usually results in the rupture of a blood vessel and severe abdominal bleeding and internal hemorrhage.

SIGNIFICANT PHYSICAL FINDINGS

1. Abdominal pain
2. Vaginal bleeding
3. Pain under the diaphragm
4. Shoulder pain
5. Urge to defecate
6. Decreased blood pressure
7. Increased pulse
8. Signs of shock: altered consciousness; rapid, weak pulse; cool, clammy skin; low blood pressure; paleness

SIGNIFICANT HISTORY

1. Missed period
2. Sudden onset of acute abdominal pain
3. Known pregnancy

PATIENT CARE

1. Administer high flow (10 to 15 LPM) of oxygen.
2. Treat for shock. If SBP below 90 and pulse above 110 or SBP below 80 regardless of pulse, apply and inflate anti-shock trousers, including abdominal chamber, if available.
3. Paramedic evaluation required; if paramedics unavailable, transport immediately.

SPECIAL CONSIDERATIONS

This is a true emergency requiring immediate treatment by paramedics or emergency room personnel.

Toxemia

DESCRIPTION

Toxemia is a condition of pregnancy due to unknown biochemical changes in the blood that cause severe vascular and neurological symptoms. It is more common with first pregnancies and starts to appear around week 24.

SIGNIFICANT PHYSICAL FINDINGS

1. Sudden weight gain
2. Swelling of face, fingers, legs, and feet
3. Blurred vision
4. Headache
5. Persistent vomiting
6. Elevated blood pressure (140/90 or higher)
7. Mental confusion, disorientation, seizures

SIGNIFICANT HISTORY

1. Diagnosis of preeclampsia
2. First pregnancy
3. More than 24 weeks pregnant
4. Last visit to obstetrician

PATIENT CARE

1. Administer moderate flow (5 to 9 LPM) of oxygen by cannula or mask.
2. If patient convulsive:
   a. Protect from injury and maintain airway.
   b. If unconscious, secure to a long backboard and position appropriately for airway maintenance.

> c. When conscious, reposition on back with head and shoulders elevated.
> 3. Minimize stimulation that might induce seizures (e.g., sirens, bright lights).
> 4. Paramedic evaluation required or transport immediately if paramedics unavailable.

SPECIAL CONSIDERATIONS

1. Toxemia is a serious complication of a pregnancy. The death rate for mothers is from 5 to 15 percent; for babies, it is about 25 percent.
2. Seizures resulting from toxemia are associated with a high death rate.

Toxic Shock Syndrome

DESCRIPTION

Sudden onset of massive septic shock. Usually accompanied by a history of tampon or diaphragm use. Although this syndrome has occurred in men and children also, it is usually seen in menstruating women.

SIGNIFICANT PHYSICAL FINDINGS AND HISTORY

1. Sudden fever, chills
2. Nausea, vomiting, diarrhea
3. Abdominal pain
4. Headaches
5. Sore throat
6. Hypertension

SPECIAL CONSIDERATIONS

1. Ensure adequate airway; be prepared to suction the airway.
2. Position the patient to allow for drainage of emesis.
3. Administer high flow (10 to 15 LPM) of oxygen.

4. Consider applying MAST.
5. Consider starting a large-bore IV.
6. Paramedic evaluation required or transport immediately.

Rape and Sexual Assault

DESCRIPTION

These are legal terms. You are treating the victim of an act of aggression who may have accompanying physical and psychological injuries. Preserve the crime scene evidence while patient care is being administered.

SIGNIFICANT PHYSICAL FINDINGS AND HISTORY

1. Maintain a nonjudgmental attitude toward the patient.
2. Talk to the patient before touching him or her.
3. Find out what the patient has done since the assault (i.e., bathed, changed clothes, etc.).

PATIENT CARE

1. Attend to any wounds or trauma.
2. Make patient as comfortable as possible.
3. Contact rape relief center in your area.
4. Do not cleanse minor wounds.
5. Do not examine the genital area. (Pad the area with a bulky-type dressing if there is obvious injury.)

SPECIAL CONSIDERATIONS

1. Your written report and comments can be used as legal evidence. Make them both as objective as possible.
2. Discuss the case only with people who are directly involved in the patient's care.

PEDIATRIC EMERGENCIES

Apnea

DESCRIPTION

"Infantile apnea" is the transient cessation of air exchange caused by a pause in respiratory effort or by obstruction in the air passages of infants under one year of age. If discovery of the infant is made soon after apnea has begun, resuscitation may be successful in restoring respirations and heart beat. There is much disagreement as to whether these "near misses" are indeed aborted SIDS events since they do not fit the current definition or even the name of the syndrome.

SIGNIFICANT PHYSICAL FINDINGS AND HISTORY

If this is true apnea and not SIDS, the infant will probably be awake and breathing, perhaps slightly cyanotic, with little evidence of any problems other than that reported by the parents or caretakers.

PATIENT CARE

1. Ensure adequate airway and respirations of 20 to 40 per minute.
2. Administer low flow (2 to 4 LPM) of oxygen (preferably humidified) by holding mask close to the infant's face if respiratory distress is evident by a respiratory rate greater than 40 or less than 20 per minute, excessive use of chest muscles, breathing through mouth or flared nostrils, or noisy respirations (wheezing, barking cough).
3. Contact infant's physician unless condition serious, requiring paramedic evaluation.

Child Abuse

DESCRIPTION

The National Center on Child Abuse and Neglect estimates that approximately 1 million children are maltreated by their parents each year. The physical and emotional impact on these children is staggering. Abuse may be physical, emotional, sexual in nature or it can be from total neglect of the child's health and well-being. Early detection and intervention is essential to the child's emotional and physical growth.

SIGNIFICANT PHYSICAL FINDINGS AND HISTORY

Each type of abuse has destructive physical and behavioral indicators that will help in identifying the abuse victim. Look for clues in child and parental behavior:

The Child

1. Apathetic; does not cry; does not seek out parent for comfort
2. Appears poorly nourished or poorly cared for
3. Evidence of multiple bruises or fractures
4. Old and new injuries
5. History of several visits to different hospitals
6. Cigarette burns, scalds on back, strap marks, welts
7. Bruises on back, buttocks, mouth

The Parent

1. Vague, evasive, conflicting stories
2. History that cannot account for injury observed
3. Long delay in seeking treatment
4. Anger, hostility, lack of appropriate concern

PATIENT CARE

1. Treat the child in the same manner as you would for any other injured child—examine carefully and stabilize.
2. *Do NOT confront or accuse the parents/suspects with your suspicions.* Such confrontation might further jeopardize the child and alienate those responsible from seeking and accepting help.
3. Anytime an EMT suspects child abuse, sexual assault, or neglect, a law enforcement officer is to be requested

to the scene. Because child abuse is considered to be an "assault" situation, and as such, a criminal offense, legal intervention is required.
4. When requesting a law enforcement officer, ask for the estimated arrival time.
    a. If a law enforcement officer is unavailable, or immediate transport is required, the child should be transported to the hospital and the officer requested to meet there.
    b. If a law enforcement officer has not arrived before the EMTs leave the hospital, the EMTs should notify the dispatcher of their return to quarters or any change in their location and request contact at new location.
5. If a law enforcement officer is unavailable, the EMTs must transport the child to the hospital and report any suspicions of child abuse to the ER staff and/or ER physician.
6. If the parents refuse to let the EMTs transport, the EMTs are to remain at the scene with the child until the law enforcement officer arrives.
7. If the injury is not serious enough to warrant a medic unit, the EMTs or an ambulance must transport the child to the nearest hospital.
8. If the EMTs are concerned about the welfare and safety of other children in the home, arrangements must be made to ensure their safety.
9. Document both subjective and objective exams; document any statements made by the parents or witnesses regarding how the injury was sustained and who was present at the time the injury was alleged to occur. All statements about the manner of injury should be documented, even if they appear to be untrue. Sign the form with name and phone number in the event further information is needed by the investigating officer.
10. If sexual abuse is evident:
    a. Minimize exam.
    b. Do not allow washing of child.
    c. Proceed with notification of law enforcement agency.
11. If suspicions of child abuse arise sometime after the event, the EMT should call 911 to make a report to a law enforcement officer.

Croup

DESCRIPTION

Croup is a viral illness most commonly seen in children between 6 months and 4 years of age resulting in swelling and narrowing of the upper airway just below the glottis.

SIGNIFICANT PHYSICAL FINDINGS

1. "Seal-like" barking cough
2. Hoarseness
3. Signs of respiratory distress: nasal flaring, tugging at the throat, retraction of the muscles around the rib cage
4. Signs of oxygen deficiency: restlessness, cyanosis
5. Fever

SIGNIFICANT HISTORY

1. Sudden or gradual onset
2. Exposure to children with similar symptoms
3. Respiratory difficulty improves during the day and worsens at night
4. Recent cold or respiratory infection

PATIENT CARE

1. Administer low flow (2 to 4 LPM) of oxygen by cannula or face mask.
2. Take child into steamy bathroom.
3. Paramedic evaluation required or transport immediately if paramedics unavailable.

SPECIAL CONSIDERATIONS

1. Because croup and epiglottitis are difficult to distinguish, any child exhibiting signs of either should be quickly transported to the hospital. Do not place anything in the child's mouth to facilitate examination. This could cause laryngospasm and complete airway obstruction.

2. The presence of drooling is strongly characteristic of epiglottitis and is not associated with croup.

Dehydration and Hypovolemia

DESCRIPTION

Bleeding is not the only cause of shock in children. Serious hypovolemia may occur due to fever, vomiting, or diarrhea. Even a small loss of fluid or blood in a child or infant can result in severe dehydration, rendering the child very sick.

SIGNIFICANT PHYSICAL FINDINGS

1. Progressive lethargy, listlessness, apathy
2. Dryness of the lips and mouth
3. Sunken eyes
4. Depressed fontanelles
5. Decreased skin turgor
6. Decreased and concentrated urine
7. Weak, rapid pulse
8. Cyanotic and/or cool extremities
9. Increased respiratory rate
10. Decreased capillary refill

SIGNIFICANT HISTORY

1. High fever
2. Recent illness with vomiting and diarrhea, reduced intake of fluids
3. Prolonged hot weather
4. Number of wet diapers per day (fewer than four to six in 24 hours is significant)

PATIENT CARE

1. Administer low flow (2 to 4 LPM) of oxygen.
2. Treat for shock. (Control bleeding.)
3. Consider pediatric MAST application.

4. Consider starting an IV.
5. Paramedic evaluation required; if paramedics unavailable, transport immediately.

SPECIAL CONSIDERATIONS

Be alert for early signs of shock. A child will often lose one-fourth of his or her blood volume before developing hypotension (apathy, listlessness, collapsed neck veins, cold, pale skin).

Epiglottitis

DESCRIPTION

Epiglottitis is a bacterial infection of the epiglottis (the lidlike structure that prevents food from entering the trachea during swallowing), resulting in severe swelling and airway obstruction. The onset of symptoms occurs very rapidly (within a few hours) and can be life threatening.

SIGNIFICANT PHYSICAL FINDINGS

1. Rapid onset of high fever
2. Severe pain on swallowing; drooling and refusal to swallow liquids because of pain
3. Child appears acutely ill
4. Child anxious and worried, but obedient
5. Child assumes a position of breathing comfort:
   a. Upright
   b. Leaning forward
   c. Chin thrust out
   d. Resists attempts to make him lie down
6. Signs of air hunger:
   a. Restlessness
   b. Rapid respiratory rate
   c. Nasal flaring
   d. Retractions
   e. Use of accessory muscles
7. Child unwilling to move

SIGNIFICANT HISTORY

1. Sudden or gradual onset
2. Exposure to other sick children
3. Recent cold or respiratory infection

PATIENT CARE

1. *Do NOT put anything into the child's mouth* under any circumstances. Such stimulation is likely to cause laryngospasm and airway obstruction.
2. Administer high flow (10 to 15 LPM) of oxygen, preferably humidified by mask.
3. Position the child upright.
4. Minimize stimulation.
5. Paramedic evaluation required; if paramedics unavailable, transport immediately.

SPECIAL CONSIDERATIONS

Because croup and epiglottitis are difficult to distinguish, any child exhibiting signs of either should be quickly evaluated by paramedics or transported to the hospital.

Febrile Seizures

DESCRIPTION

A febrile seizure is a convulsion brought on by a high fever, usually over 104°F. The seizure usually occurs within the first few hours of the fever. Ninety-eight percent of children experiencing a febrile seizure will outgrow them, and only 2 percent develop epilepsy.

SIGNIFICANT PHYSICAL FINDINGS AND HISTORY

1. Fever, stiff neck
2. Recent illness or infection
3. Tonic–clonic seizure activity
4. Postictal disorientation, sleepiness, unconsciousness

PATIENT CARE

1. If patient still seizing:
   a. Call a medic unit.
   b. Protect patient from injury.
   c. Administer moderate flow (5 to 9 LPM) of oxygen by mask.
2. If seizing stopped:
   a. Evaluate for predisposing factors.
   b. Take rectal temperature.
   c. Remove all types of clothing, but keep lightly covered if rectal temperature above 101° (38.3°C).
   d. Call for paramedic evaluation, or transport to hospital.

SPECIAL CONSIDERATIONS

1. Sponging the child in the field is ineffective and should not be performed.
2. All seizures other than febrile require transport and further medical evaluation.
3. Antipyretics (aspirin or acetominophen) should be administered only with instructions from base hospital or private physician.

Poisonings

DESCRIPTION

A poison is any liquid, solid, or gas that impairs health or causes death when it is introduced into the body or onto the skin surface. Approximately 90 percent of all poisoning cases involve children. Poisonings can be accidental or intentional and can result from the ingestion of substances; inhalation of dust, vapors, gases; injection from hypodermic needles or insect/snake bites; or absorption of substances from the skin.

SIGNIFICANT PHYSICAL FINDINGS

The signs and symptoms of any poisoning will vary depending on the substance and mechanism of entry. The most common ones for substance ingestion are:

1. Nausea, vomiting, diarrhea
2. Severe abdominal pain and cramps
3. Slowed respiration
4. Low blood pressure
5. Excessive salivation or sweating
6. Skin discoloration around the mouth
7. Characteristic odors such as kerosene, gasoline, turpentine
8. Contents of a drug bottle spilled out and not accounted for
9. Unconsciousness
10. Convulsions

SIGNIFICANT HISTORY

1. Previous history of poisoning/accidental ingestions
2. Exposure to possible sources
3. Medical history: medications, disease, suicidal tendencies
4. Action taken by bystanders: vomiting induced, ipecac administered, antidotes given, and so on

---

PATIENT CARE

1. In cases of breathing difficulties, convulsions, or unconsciousness:
   a. Assess and support ABCs.
   b. Administer oxygen appropriate to condition.
   c. Request paramedic evaluation or transport immediately to nearest emergency room.
   d. Transport with head elevated and lying on either side.
   e. If unconscious, secure patient on long backboard and position appropriately for airway maintenance.
2. For external contamination:
   a. Protect medical personnel.
   b. Remove contaminated clothing.
   c. Flush contaminated skin and eyes with copious amounts of water.
3. Read the label on the poison container to determine ingredients.
4. Call the base hospital of your provider group.
5. Monitor vital signs.

Sudden Infant Death Syndrome

DESCRIPTION

Sudden infant death syndrome (SIDS) is the sudden and unexpected death of a seemingly healthy infant which remains unexplained even after a careful autopsy. SIDS is the leading cause of death in infants between 2 weeks and 1 year of age.

SIGNIFICANT PHYSICAL FINDINGS

1. Frothy drainage from nose/mouth
2. Cooling/rigor mortis
3. Lividity—settling of blood
4. Appears well developed

SIGNIFICANT HISTORY

1. Child usually asleep prior to being found
2. Illness within last 2 weeks
3. Premature or low birth weight
4. One of twins or triplets
5. Previous family history of SIDS or apnea (prolonged breathing pauses)

PATIENT CARE

1. Initiate CPR according to protocols.
2. Provide support to family; suggest that family call the SIDS support group.
3. Paramedic evaluation required or transport immediately if medics unavailable.

SPECIAL CONSIDERATIONS

1. SIDS rarely occurs during the first few weeks of life; peak incidence is between 2 and 4 months; rare after 6 months.
2. SIDS is more common in boys than in girls.

3. SIDS occurs at a higher rate:
   a. Among blacks and American Indians than in whites and orientals
   b. In low socioeconomic families
   c. In premature and low-birth-weight infants
   d. In twins and triplets
   e. In families with a history of SIDS or apnea
4. Emotional support is strongly needed for the parents.

RESPIRATORY EMERGENCIES

Asthma

DESCRIPTION

Asthma is characterized by episodic, acute attacks of bronchospasms in which the airways become swollen, constricted, and filled with mucus. Allergens, chemical and environmental irritants, emotional stress, and infection can trigger an attack. Between episodes the patient is symptom-free.

SIGNIFICANT PHYSICAL FINDINGS
1. Extreme difficulty breathing; patient tense and frightened
2. Upright position, leaning forward
3. Wheezing audible even without stethoscope
4. Use of accessory muscles
5. Quiet lung sounds if attack severe, indicating little movement of air
6. Rapid pulse rate
7. Diaphoresis

SIGNIFICANT HISTORY
1. Previous attacks
2. Exposure to irritants
3. Recent illness or infection
4. Medical history
5. Allergies

PATIENT CARE

1. Be calm and reassuring.
2. Administer low flow (2 to 4 LPM) of oxygen by cannula or face mask.
3. Keep patient sitting upright.
4. Monitor vital signs, respiratory status, and level of consciousness.
5. Assist patient in taking prescribed asthma medication.
6. Request paramedic evaluation if indicated by significant physical findings as listed in Appendix 12.

SPECIAL CONSIDERATIONS

1. A sleepy asthmatic with quiet breath sounds is a true medical emergency in need of immediate intervention.
2. *Status asthmaticus* is a severe, prolonged asthmatic attack that does not respond to the usual medications and *can be fatal,* requiring urgent paramedic care and transport.

Chronic Obstructive Pulmonary Disease

DESCRIPTION

The two most common chronic obstructive pulmonary diseases (COPD) are emphysema and chronic bronchitis. Both result in destructive changes in the lung that lead to progressive dyspnea and debilitation. Patients with COPD have little respiratory reserve, such that a minor respiratory illness can become life threatening.

SIGNIFICANT PHYSICAL FINDINGS

1. Respiratory distress
2. Confused and agitated, or sleepy and lethargic
3. Cyanosis
4. Rapid pulse
5. Breathing in puffs through pursed lips
6. Use of accessory muscles to breathe
7. Wheezing

8. Cannot tolerate lying flat
9. Diaphoresis
10. Chest pain
11. Productive cough

SIGNIFICANT HISTORY

1. Chronic dyspnea, recently worse
2. Current or past heavy smoker
3. Recent respiratory infection or illness
4. Changes in the amount and color of sputum
5. On home oxygen
6. History of orthopnea or awakening at night in respiratory distress
7. Number of pillows they sleep with at night
8. Medical history
9. Current medications

PATIENT CARE

1. Maintain an open airway.
2. Keep patient sitting upright.
3. Administer low flow (2 to 4 LPM) of oxygen by nasal cannula, or high flow (10 to 15 LPM) by mask if in acute respiratory distress (see page 98). Have bag-valve mask device readily available.
4. Prepare to assist ventilations with bag-valve-mask if respirations become depressed, fewer than eight per minute or level of consciousness decreases.
5. Apply ECG monitor.
6. Loosen tight clothing.
7. Encourage patient to cough up sputum.
8. Keep patient warm but not overheated.
9. Consider an IV of D_5W KVO.
10. Request paramedic evaluation if indicated by significant physical findings as listed in Appendix 12.

SPECIAL CONSIDERATIONS

1. Never withhold oxygen therapy from a patient in respiratory distress, even if there is a history of COPD. Prepare to assist if respirations become depressed.
2. It is sometimes difficult to get these patients to accept a mask because of their severe distress and breathing difficulty. Explain to them that they will receive more oxygen if they wear the mask.

Hyperventilation Syndrome

DESCRIPTION

Hyperventilation syndrome occurs primarily in anxious young patients as a result of rapid breathing in excess of 20 breaths per minute. Causes include emotional stress, anxiety, and physical exertion. Patients are usually unaware that they are breathing abnormally.

SIGNIFICANT PHYSICAL FINDINGS

1. Young, anxious patient near panic
2. Rapid respirations
3. Flushed skin
4. Fainting
5. Carpopedal spasms or a contorted position of the hands in which the fingers are flexed like claws and the thumbs curl in toward the palm
6. Normal breath sounds
7. Numbness or tingling around the mouth, hands, and feet
8. Dizziness, lightheadedness
9. Blurring of vision
10. Pounding of the heart

SIGNIFICANT HISTORY

1. Experiencing family or personal crisis
2. Prone to anxiety
3. Previous experience with rapid breathing
4. Medical history
5. Current medications

PATIENT CARE

1. Maintain a calm and reassuring approach.
2. Have patient breathe into a paper bag.
3. Have patient evaluated by private physician after episode.
4. Request paramedic evaluation if indicated by significant physical findings as listed in Appendix 12.

SPECIAL CONSIDERATIONS

Not every patient who is breathing deeply or rapidly is actually hyperventilating. Diabetics with metabolic acidosis or acute alcohol intoxication can exhibit similar symptoms, but such cases are more serious, requiring different treatment and care.

Pneumonia

DESCRIPTION

Pneumonia is an acute disease characterized by inflammation of the lungs, resulting in the accumulation of fluid or pus in the alveoli and disruption of the oxygenation of the blood. It can be caused by bacteria, viruses, aspirated vomitus, or inhaled chemical agents.

SIGNIFICANT PHYSICAL FINDINGS

1. Cough; dark sputum
2. Appearing acutely ill
3. Fever with hot, dry skin
4. Respiratory distress
5. Rhonchi or noisy, rattling lung sounds
6. Rapid respiratory rate (above 30 per minute)

SIGNIFICANT HISTORY

1. Sudden onset of fever and shaking chills
2. Chest pain on inspiration
3. Shortness of breath
4. Elderly or debilitated patients
5. Recent illness

PATIENT CARE

1. Administer low flow (2 to 4 LPM) of oxygen by nasal cannula.
2. Position patient in semireclining position.
3. Apply ECG monitor.
4. Request paramedic evaluation if indicated by significant physical findings as listed in Appendix 12.
5. Consider an IV of D_5W KVO.

SPECIAL CONSIDERATIONS

Pneumonia can become life threatening for elderly, debilitated, or chronically ill people, requiring urgent care and transport to the hospital.

Pneumothorax (spontaneous)

DESCRIPTION

The presence of air within the pleural sac surrounding the lungs is defined as a pneumothorax usually resulting from direct injury to the lung. A spontaneous pneumothorax can occur without injury and is typically seen in people who have scattered weak areas in their lung tissue that rupture or tear. Commonly seen in patients with chronic obstructive lung diseases.

SIGNIFICANT PHYSICAL FINDINGS

1. Respiratory distress, and respiratory rate above 30 per minute
2. Absent or decreased lung sounds over affected lung
3. Deviation or shift of trachea if severe opposite the side of the affected lung

SIGNIFICANT HISTORY

1. Sudden sharp chest pain
2. Shortness of breath
3. History of respiratory disease

> **PATIENT CARE**
>
> 1. Administer moderate flow of oxygen (5 to 9 LPM) by cannula or face mask.
> 2. Keep patient sitting up.
> 3. Apply ECG monitor.
> 4. Paramedic evaluation required; if paramedics unavailable, transport immediately.
> 5. Consider starting an IV.

Pulmonary Edema

DESCRIPTION

Pulmonary edema is the accumulation of fluids in the lungs as a result of failure of the left side of the heart to pump blood effectively, or direct damage to the alveoli from toxic gas or smoke inhalation, near-drowning, aspiration pneumonia, narcotic overdose, or high altitude. The presence of fluid in the alveoli impairs gas exchange of oxygen and carbon dioxide resulting in respiratory distress and possibly arrest.

SIGNIFICANT PHYSICAL FINDINGS

1. Respiratory distress
2. Rapid respiratory rate, greater than 30 per minute
3. Confusion, agitation, combativeness
4. Rapid pulse rate, elevated blood pressure
5. Frothy pink sputum
6. Cyanosis
7. Rales and wheezes
8. Diaphoresis

SIGNIFICANT HISTORY

1. Severe shortness of breath that worsens when lying flat
2. Possible chest pain
3. Chronic hypertension or heart disease

4. History of congestive heart failure (CHF) or COPD
5. History of near-drowning
6. History of narcotic overdose

PATIENT CARE

1. Administer moderate to high flow (5 to 15 LPM) of oxygen as tolerated by patient. Have bag-valve mask available for use.
2. Keep patient upright.
3. Apply ECG monitor.
4. Consider IV.
5. Paramedic evaluation required or transport immediately if paramedics unavailable.

Pulmonary Embolism

DESCRIPTION

A pulmonary embolism is the sudden obstruction of a pulmonary artery by a blood clot or foreign body (air bubbles, fat particles) blocking the flow of blood and resulting in hypoxia, severe hypotension, and possible death. Blood clots are formed due to prolonged bedrest, inactivity, inflamed veins, or birth control pills. Fat particles released from severe fractures or air bubbles from an open neck wound can also cause a pulmonary embolism.

SIGNIFICANT PHYSICAL FINDINGS

1. Severe respiratory distress and rapid respirations (greater than 30 per minute)
2. Rapid pulse: above 100 to 110
3. Hypotension
4. Associated signs of shock: altered consciousness; rapid, weak pulse; cool, clammy skin; low blood pressure; paleness
5. Continued cyanosis even after oxygen administration
6. Rapid respirations in the elderly for no apparent reason

SIGNIFICANT HISTORY

1. Prolonged bedrest, inactivity
2. Thrombophlebitis
3. On birth control pills
4. Recent surgery or bone fractures
5. Acute onset of shortness of breath
6. Localized, sharp chest pain

PATIENT CARE

1. Administer high flow (10 to 15 LPM) of oxygen by nonrebreathing mask; be prepared to initiate CPR. Assist respirations as needed with bag-valve mask.
2. Position patient for comfort.
3. Treat for shock if SBP below 90 and pulse above 110, or SBP below 80 regardless of pulse; apply and inflate antishock trousers if available.
4. Paramedic evaluation required; if paramedics unavailable, transport immediately.

SPECIAL CONSIDERATION

Without a good history, pulmonary embolism is hard to diagnose. Treat the symptoms.

Respiratory Distress

DESCRIPTION

Respiratory distress can occur any time that airflow or the exchange of oxygen and carbon monoxide is impaired. The body attempts to overcome this impairment by increasing the rate and depth of respirations. Unless corrected, the continuing decrease in oxygen and increase in carbon dioxide levels depress the respiratory control center, slowing respirations and resulting in unconsciousness and ultimately respiratory and cardiac arrest.

SIGNIFICANT PHYSICAL FINDINGS

1. Altered level of awareness; dizziness, fainting, restlessness, anxiety, confusion, combativeness; unconsciousness
2. Respiratory rate less than 8 or greater than 30 per minute
3. Flaring nostrils
4. Strained intercostal and abdominal muscles
5. Retraction of neck muscles
6. Pursed lips
7. Noisy respirations: wheezing, rales, rattling
8. Numbness or tingling in hands and feet
9. Cyanosis

SIGNIFICANT HISTORY

1. Complaint of shortness of breath or difficulty getting enough air
2. Chronic respiratory or cardiac disease
3. History of COPD, emphysema, bronchitis
4. History of smoking
5. Home oxygen use
6. Recent illness or upper respiratory infections
7. Recent hospitalizations
8. Current medications
9. Allergies

PATIENT CARE

1. Administer high flow (10 to 15 LPM) of oxygen by face mask or nonrebreather.
2. Prepare to assist ventilations with bag-valve-mask if respirations become seriously depressed or stop.
3. Apply ECG monitor.
4. Reassure patients; talk to them to help reduce their anxiety and sense of panic.
5. Position as patient is comfortable with head elevated.
6. Consider an IV of D_5W KVO.
7. Paramedic evaluation required; if paramedics unavailable, transport immediately.

SHOCK

General Protocols for Shock

DESCRIPTION

Shock is the result of circulatory failure leading to an inadequate flow of oxygenated blood to the body organs. Shock can occur by several mechanisms:

1. Severe allergic reaction (*anaphylactic shock*) from exposure to a foreign substance, insect stings or bites, blood infusions, food, or desensitizing antigens. Death can occur in minutes from airway obstruction or shock as a result of peripheral vasodilation.
2. Failure of the heart (*cardiogenic shock*) caused by damage to the heart muscle, pericardial tamponade, tension pneumothorax, or arrhythmias leading to an inadequate output of blood from the heart.
3. Decreased blood or fluid volume (*hypovolemic shock*) resulting from internal or external bleeding, burns or dehydration (from vomiting, diarrhea, inadequate water intake).
4. Increased vascular space (*neurogenic shock*) as a result of injury to the spinal cord or drug overdose. The blood vessels in the extremities dilate and blood pools, decreasing the amount of blood returning to the heart.
5. Decreased oxygenation (*respiratory shock*) resulting from inadequate breathing, pulmonary embolism, or respiratory arrest due to spinal cord injury, obstruction of the airways, or chest trauma.
6. Bacterial infection of the blood (*septic shock*) in which the body reacts violently to toxins released by the bacteria, resulting in dilation of blood vessels and leakage of fluid from damaged capillaries.

SIGNIFICANT PHYSICAL FINDINGS

1. Altered level of consciousness: restlessness, anxiety, confusion
2. Vital signs:
    a. Weak and thready pulse; pulse rate above 110
    b. Gradual and steady drop in BP to 90/60 or less
    c. Respirations shallow and fast

3. Skin: cold, clammy, moist; profuse sweating; extreme pallor or cyanosis
4. External bleeding
5. Signs of trauma, evidence of blunt injury
6. Signs of heart failure: distended neck veins, wet breath sounds
7. Nausea, vomiting
8. Intense thirst

SIGNIFICANT HISTORY

1. Onset can be sudden or gradual; precipitating cause can be a traumatic or a nontraumatic event
2. Associate symptoms: chest pain, abdominal pain, itching, hives, facial or peripheral edema, dizziness on standing
3. History: fever and chills, recent surgery or illness, significant medical diseases
4. Current medications
5. Known allergies

PATIENT CARE

1. Maintain open airway. Manage respirations as needed.
2. Administer high flow (10 to 15 LPM) of oxygen by nonrebreather mask or bag-valve-mask device.
3. Control obvious bleeding.
4. Splint all fractures.
5. If SBP below 90 and pulse above 110 or SBP below 80 regardless of pulse, apply and inflate medical antishock trousers if available.
    a. *Anaphylactic shock:* Assist the person in administering injectable or oral antiallergic medication.
    b. *Neurogenic shock:* Stabilize neck and immobilize on long backboard.
    c. *Cardiogenic shock:* Use of the medical antishock trousers is absolutely contraindicated.
6. Apply ECG monitor.
7. Lay patient flat and elevate legs on backboard (if immobilized) to 30° or 12 inches. Apply and inflate medical antishock trousers if available and not contraindicated.

8. Get patient off ground and out of weather. Cover patient to avoid excess heat loss, but do not overwrap.
9. Consider starting an IV.
10. Give nothing by mouth.
11. Have suction available.
12. Monitor vital signs and level of consciousness.
13. Paramedic evaluation required; if paramedics unavailable, transport immediately.

SPECIAL CONSIDERATION

To prevent irreversible shock and eventual death, adequate blood flow must be restored as soon as possible. Treatment is aimed at controlling bleeding, elevating the blood pressure, and administering high concentrations of oxygen.

Anaphylactic Shock

SIGNIFICANT PHYSICAL FINDINGS

1. Difficulty breathing, respiratory distress, wheezing
2. Itching, hives
3. Flushing around the face and chest
4. Blueness around the lips
5. Swelling of the face and tongue
6. Paleness
7. Weak, rapid pulse
8. Low blood pressure
9. Dizziness
10. Anxiety
11. Altered level of consciousness
12. Painful, squeezing sensation in the chest
13. Nausea, vomiting
14. Abdominal cramps
15. Incontinence of urine and stool
16. Seizures

SIGNIFICANT HISTORY

1. Known allergies
2. Previous allergic reaction and severity

3. Recent exposure to possible substances
4. Time since onset of symptoms

PATIENT CARE

1. Maintain open airway. Assist respirations as needed.
2. Administer high flow (10 to 15 LPM) of oxygen by nonrebreather mask.
3. Assist patient in administering injectable or oral medication, if available (Special Consideration 2).
4. Lay patient flat and elevate legs.
5. Apply ECG monitor.
6. If SBP below 90 and pulse above 110, or SBP below 80 regardless of pulse, apply and inflate all chambers of medical antishock trousers if available.
7. Consider starting an IV of normal saline with large-bore needle.
8. Paramedic evaluation required; if paramedics unavailable, transport immediately.

SPECIAL CONSIDERATIONS

1. Anaphylaxis is an extreme emergency since cardiac arrest can occur within seconds. Do not delay treatment or transport.
2. Epinephrine or adrenalin is the medication often prescribed to patients with known serious allergies. Administered by injection, pill, or inhaler, this drug can reduce the severity of associated bronchospasm and can be lifesaving. EMTs may assist patient in administering these medications.

Cardiogenic Shock

SIGNIFICANT PHYSICAL FINDINGS

1. Rapid or slow pulse
2. Neck vein distension
3. Wet lung sounds
4. Increased, labored respirations
5. Low blood pressure: below 90/60

SIGNIFICANT HISTORY

1. Chest pain
2. SOB and respiratory distress
3. Recent myocardial infarction or illness
4. Evidence of chest trauma
5. Medical history: cardiac or respiratory disease, hypertension, surgeries, hospitalizations
6. Current medications

PATIENT CARE

1. Administer high flow (10 to 15 LPM) of oxygen by nonrebreather mask and prepare to assist breathing with a bag-valve mask.
2. Sit patient upright or in position of comfort.
3. Apply ECG monitor.
4. Consider starting an IV.
5. Use of the medical antishock trousers is *absolutely* contraindicated.
6. Paramedic evaluation required; if paramedics unavailable, transport immediately.

Hypovolemic Shock

SIGNIFICANT PHYSICAL FINDINGS

1. Cool, moist (clammy) skin
2. Intense thirst
3. Rapid, weak pulse
4. Paleness
5. Low blood pressure: below 90/60
6. Postural hypotension (pulse rise above 20 or systolic BP drop above 20 mmHg)
7. Obvious bleeding
8. Signs of internal bleeding (i.e., rigid abdomen)
9. Decreased capillary refill

SIGNIFICANT HISTORY

1. Blunt or penetrating trauma to chest, abdomen, pelvis, thigh
2. Burns
3. Prolonged vomiting/diarrhea
4. Bloody, "coffee-like" emesis
5. Bloody or tarry stools
6. Medical history: diabetes, gastric ulcers, alcohol use, surgeries
7. Current medications

PATIENT CARE

1. Administer high flow (10 to 15 LPM) of oxygen by nonrebreather mask.
2. Control obvious bleeding.
3. Splint all fractures.
4. If SBP below 90 and pulse above 110, or SBP below 80 regardless of pulse, apply and inflate antishock trousers if available.
5. Elevate legs (if MAST unavailable) or backboard (if immobilized) to 30° or 12 inches.
6. Consider starting an IV.
7. Conserve body heat, but do not overwrap.
8. Give nothing by mouth.
9. Paramedic evaluation required; if paramedics unavailable, transport immediately.
10. Repeat vital signs frequently.

SPECIAL CONSIDERATIONS

1. Do not be misled by the blood pressure since this may remain normal as long as the patient is lying flat. The pulse will give an early indication of possible problems.
2. Keeping the patient too warm may cause peripheral vasodilitation, worsening the patient's hypovolemia.

Neurogenic Shock

SIGNIFICANT PHYSICAL FINDINGS

1. Low blood pressure (below 90/60), with slow, regular pulse
2. Warm and dry skin
3. Cuts and bruises to the head, face, neck, or back, suggesting trauma
4. Priapism or sustained erection in the male patient
5. Loss of sensation below the nipple line

SIGNIFICANT HISTORY

1. Evidence of trauma
2. Numbness or paralysis
3. Emotional distress, severe pain
4. History of drug abuse

PATIENT CARE

1. Administer high flow (10 to 15 LPM) of oxygen by nonrebreather mask.
2. Prepare backboard and position antishock trousers for possible inflation if available.
3. Properly immobilize when positioned on the backboard.
4. If SBP below 90 and pulse above 110, or SBP below 80 regardless of pulse, inflate antishock trousers if available.
5. Consider an IV.
6. Paramedic evaluation required; if paramedics unavailable, transport immediately.

SPECIAL CONSIDERATIONS

1. Emotional distress, severe pain, or fright (often referred to as psychogenic shock) can produce the same findings. This type of shock quickly passes once the patient is lying flat.
2. Neurogenic shock is self-initiating and usually responds to leg elevation or inflation of medical antishock trousers.

3. If shock is severe, consider internal injuries of the chest, abdomen, or pelvis, where blood loss can be significant.
4. Trendelenberg or head-down position causes the abdominal contents to push on the diaphragm, decreasing effectiveness of respirations. Simple leg elevation or application of MAST is preferred.

Respiratory Shock

SIGNIFICANT PHYSICAL FINDINGS

1. Restlessness, agitation, combativeness due to hypoxemia or low oxygen
2. Rapid respiratory rate: above 30 per minute
3. Labored respirations, use of accessory muscles
4. Rapid or slow and irregular pulse
5. Hypotension
6. Cyanosis

SIGNIFICANT HISTORY

1. Evidence of traumatic injury
2. Medical history: recent illness or surgery, medical problems
3. Current medications

PATIENT CARE

1. Administer high flow (10 to 15 LPM) of oxygen with nonrebreather mask or bag-valve-mask device.
2. Support respirations as indicated; prepare to initiate CPR.
3. Treat life-threatening injuries (i.e., pneumothorax, flail chest).
4. If SBP below 90 and pulse above 110, or SBP below 80 regardless of pulse, apply and inflate antishock trousers if available. Monitor respirations closely.
5. Consider an IV.
6. Paramedic evaluation required; if paramedics unavailable, transport immediately.

Septic Shock

SIGNIFICANT PHYSICAL FINDINGS

1. Fever and chills
2. Hot, dry, and flushed skin
3. Nausea
4. Low blood pressure: below 90/60
5. Rapid heart rate: above 110

SIGNIFICANT HISTORY

1. Feeling of general malaise
2. Medical history: urinary tract infections, pregnancies, recent miscarriage or abortion, diabetes, cancer
3. Current medications
4. IV drug abuse

PATIENT CARE

1. Administer high flow (10 to 15 LPM) of oxygen by nonrebreathing mask or bag-valve mask device.
2. Treat for shock. If SBP below 90 and pulse above 110, or SBP below 80 regardless of pulse, apply and inflate medical antishock trousers if available.
3. Consider starting an IV.
4. Paramedic evaluation required or transport immediately if paramedics unavailable.

TRAUMATIC INJURIES

Traumatic Cardiopulmonary Arrest (Presumed Exsanguination)

DESCRIPTION

Patient has a witnessed cardiac arrest due to trauma. This patient is presumed to have suffered exsanguinating blood loss. Patients who are observed to have some signs of life have the best chance for resuscitation.

SIGNIFICANT PHYSICAL FINDINGS

1. Unconscious, unresponsive
2. Pulseless, breathless
3. Pale mottled color
4. Noncranial penetrating or blunt trauma

SIGNIFICANT HISTORY

Someone witnessed signs of life after the trauma.

PATIENT CARE

Every act should be performed while moving this patient toward surgery.

1. Establish the airway using cervical spine precautions.
2. Administer CPR.
3. Immobilize on a backboard with MAST suit in place.
4. Control obvious external bleeding and inflate MAST.
5. Hyperventilate using 100 percent oxygen.
6. Transport.
7. Consider starting two large-bore IVs enroute.

SPECIAL CONSIDERATION

These patients must be moved as quickly as possible to a trauma center that has the ability to perform surgical repair of the injury.

Abdominal Trauma

DESCRIPTION

The abdomen contains both hollow and solid organs. The rupture or perforation of hollow organs of the digestive system spills contents into the peritoneal cavity, causing inflammation. Rupture or perforation of a solid organ such as the liver, spleen, or pancreas can result in severe bleeding. Patients involved in traumatic accidents should be evaluated for possible abdominal injuries.

SIGNIFICANT PHYSICAL FINDINGS

1. Rigid, distended, tender abdomen
2. Guarding
3. Fetal position
4. Radiation of pain to shoulder or lower back as with kidney injuries
5. Signs of shock: altered consciousness; rapid, weak pulse; cool, clammy skin; low blood pressure; paleness
6. Nausea or vomiting, sometimes bloody vomitus
7. Evisceration and protrusion of abdominal contents
8. Obvious lacerations and puncture wounds
9. Bloody urine

SIGNIFICANT HISTORY

1. Mechanism of injury
2. Blunt or penetrating trauma to abdomen
3. Description of pain

PATIENT CARE

1. Control external bleeding and dress all open wounds.
2. Administer oxygen as condition indicates.
3. Treat for shock. If SBP below 90 and pulse above 110, or SBP below 80 regardless of pulse, apply and inflate anti-shock trousers if available.
4. Consider starting an IV.
5. Apply a sheet of saran wrap followed by a dry, bulky dressing over evisceration.
6. Stabilize impaled objects with bulky dressings which are bandaged in place. Do not attempt to remove.
7. If patient not in shock, place on back with legs flexed at the knees for comfort.
8. Be alert for vomiting. Have suction available.
9. Request paramedic evaluation if indicated by significant physical findings as listed in Appendix 12.

SPECIAL CONSIDERATIONS

1. Penetrating abdominal wounds, such as those caused by a bullet, are associated with wounds in adjacent areas of the body. A complete patient survey is essential to determine extent of injuries.
2. Some patients show some relief of abdominal pain when allowed to hold a pillow or other soft, bulky object against the abdomen.

Amputations

DESCRIPTION

Amputation is the complete severing of an appendage, such as fingers, toes, hands, feet, or entire limbs, leaving jagged skin and bone edges. Often, massive bleeding results from exposed blood vessels. With proper care of the injured extremity and severed part, reimplantation is possible.

SIGNIFICANT PHYSICAL FINDINGS

1. Excessive bleeding
2. Exposed bone and tissue
3. Signs of shock: altered consciousness; weak, rapid pulse; cool, clammy skin; low blood pressure; paleness
4. Associated trauma to other body parts

SIGNIFICANT HISTORY

1. Time and mechanism of injury
2. Evidence of other traumatic injuries
3. Condition of severed part
4. Medical history and current medications
5. Any bleeding problems

PATIENT CARE

1. Control bleeding at site of amputation with direct pressure or pressure points.
2. Cover stump gently with sterile dressing.

3. Elevate extremity after bleeding is controlled.
4. Consider starting an IV with a large-bore needle.
5. Wrap completely amputated parts in sterile dressings and soak in sterile normal saline solution. Place in watertight container (specimen cup, plastic bag) and place container on ice.
6. Transport the part with the patient.
7. Request paramedic evaluation if indicated by significant physical findings as listed in Appendix 12.

SPECIAL CONSIDERATIONS

1. Rapid transport of patient and severed part is critical to the success of reimplantation. If transport is delayed, consider sending amputated part ahead to be surgically prepared.
2. Do not use dry ice to preserve severed parts.
3. Partial amputations should be dressed and splinted in alignment with extremity and elevated with the extremity.

Chest Injuries

DESCRIPTION

Injuries to the chest can result from blunt trauma, penetrating objects, or compression, such as that occurring when the chest is squeezed between the steering wheel and seat. Chest injuries are classified as open or closed. Open injuries exist when the skin is broken or the chest wall is penetrated. Closed injuries are sustained through blunt trauma and compression, causing internal damage without evidence of external injury. Trauma to the chest can result in soft tissue injuries, fractured ribs, flail chest, spontaneous or tension pneumothorax, cardiac tamponade, abdominal injuries, tearing of the major blood vessels, and traumatic asphyxia.

SIGNIFICANT PHYSICAL FINDINGS

1. Obvious open wounds
2. Unequal chest expansion
3. Unequal breath sounds
4. Sucking sounds with each respiration

5. Pain at the site of injury
6. Painful breathing
7. Difficulty breathing
8. Rapid, weak pulse, indicating hypovolemic or respiratory shock
9. Low blood pressure
10. Cyanosis, indicating lack of oxygen
11. Distended neck veins
12. Deviated trachea
13. Marked cyanosis of head, neck, and shoulders
14. Bulging and bloodshot eyes
15. Swelling of the lips and tongue

SIGNIFICANT HISTORY

1. Mechanism of injury and estimate of force involved
2. Medical history, current medical problems
3. Medications
4. Medical identification tag

PATIENT CARE

1. Maintain open airway and adequate respirations, assist as needed.
2. Administer moderate to high flow (5 to 15 LPM) of oxygen as indicated.
3. Control bleeding.
4. Treat for shock. If SBP below 90 and pulse above 110, or SBP below 80 regardless of pulse, apply and inflate antishock trousers if available.
5. Take BP in both arms.
6. Consider starting large-bore IV.
7. For sucking chest wounds, cover with occlusive dressing (saran wrap, aluminum foil, or Vaseline gauze) as the patient exhales. Place gauze bandage over occlusive dressing and tape the top and sides only, leaving the

bottom side open. Transport injured side down. If respiratory status deteriorates, open occlusive dressing briefly to see if air escapes under pressure.

8. Stabilize rib fractures by placing the patient's arm on the affected side against the chest and wrap three cravats around arm and chest; support arm with swathe. If patient unstable, stabilize with patient positioned on injured side.
9. Stabilize flail chest by applying sandbag or pad over site and tape to both sides of the chest. Pressure with one hand over the affected area may offer enough splinting for temporary purposes.
10. Stabilize impaled objects.
11. For suspected myocardial contusion (bruised myocardium) apply ECG monitor to the patient during transport to the hospital.
12. Evaluate for abdominal injuries possibly caused by trauma to the lower chest; check for exit wound with gunshot injuries.
13. Apply ECG monitor.
14. Request paramedic evaluation if indicated by significant physical findings as listed in Appendix 12.

SPECIAL CONSIDERATIONS

1. Chest injuries sufficient to cause respiratory distress are commonly associated with significant blood loss. Look for signs of hypovolemic shock, and be prepared to assist respirations with a bag-valve mask.
2. Major complications of chest injury are usually so severe as to require advanced medical procedures available only in the hospital. Rapid transport while continuing basic life support measures may be all the EMT can provide to keep the patient alive.
3. Traumatic asphyxia results from the sudden compression of the chest. This is a life-threatening emergency and requires immediate transport with artificial ventilation and 100 percent oxygen. Signs and symptoms include:
   a. Marked cyanosis of the head, neck, and shoulders
   b. Bulging and bloodshot eyes
   c. Swollen tongue and lips

Facial Injuries

DESCRIPTION

Facial injuries resulting from trauma can involve soft tissue of the face, ears, nose, and eyes or facial bones. Sufficient trauma to the face can also result in injuries to the head, brain, neck, or spine. A complete secondary survey is essential to detect other serious injuries.

SIGNIFICANT PHYSICAL FINDINGS

1. Obvious open wounds
2. Severe bruising, swelling, and pain
3. Discoloration, particularly around eyes
4. Deformity
5. Loose teeth
6. Bleeding in the mouth
7. Loose bone segments
8. Increased salivation
9. Inability to swallow or talk
10. Limited jaw movement
11. Impaired vision, especially double vision
12. Bloody or clear fluid drainage from ears or nose
13. Sunken eye sockets
14. Bulging eyeballs

SIGNIFICANT HISTORY

1. Mechanism of injury
2. Any exposure to toxic chemicals
3. Current medical problems and medications

PATIENT CARE

Face

1. Ensure an open and clear airway.
   a. Check the mouth and throat for loose objects or blood.
   b. Have suction ready and available.

2. Assist with ventilations and administer oxygen as condition indicates.
3. Control bleeding with as little pressure as possible so as not to displace fractures.
4. Check level of consciousness and note changes in behavior indicating possible brain injury.
5. Major facial injuries are often associated with spinal injuries. Immobilize if there is any question.
6. Position the patient so that blood will drain out of the mouth.
   a. Patients with bleeding facial injuries should be transported on their side with head down for drainage.
   b. Patients who are not bleeding should be transported with their heads and upper body elevated.
   c. Patients immobilized on backboard may require positioning board on its side to allow for drainage and airway maintenance.
7. Dress and bandage open wounds.
   a. Cover exposed nerves, tendons, or blood vessels with a dry, sterile dressing.
   b. Cover completely or partially avulsed areas with dry, sterile dressing.
   c. Cover lacerations and abrasions with dry, sterile dressings.
8. Save any avulsed parts (ears, nose, broken teeth, or dentures) in the following manner:
   a. Wrap in a sterile dressing and place in a sterile bag or container and soak in normal saline.
   b. Place bag or container on ice.
   c. Transport part with patient.
9. Keep patient quiet.
10. Monitor airway, vital signs, and level of consciousness.

Eyes

1. Check pupils and position of eyes.
2. Irrigate chemical burns for 20 minutes with sterile or plain water.
3. Cover lacerations of the eyelid with saline-moistened eye patches. Do not attempt to force open.
4. Care for avulsed or protruding eyeballs.
   a. Cover the eyeball or socket with protective cup.

    b. Bandage both eyes.
    c. Position patient with face up and head immobilized.
5. Stabilize impaled objects.
6. Leave contact lenses in place.
7. Leave blood clots undisturbed.

Nose

1. Maintain a clear and open airway.
2. Allow clear fluid from the nose to drain freely.
3. Avoid using pressure to stop nosebleed if bleeding is the result of traumatic injury.
4. Apply ice compress to fractured nose.
5. Leave foreign objects in place—do not attempt to remove.
6. Position patient with head and shoulders elevated to allow for drainage.

Mouth, Jaw, Cheeks

1. Protect the airway; use suction drainage as needed.
2. Firmly apply wraps to keep a fractured jaw stable during transport unless patient is bleeding from the mouth or vomiting.
3. Remove impaled objects of the cheek and pack the inside with a dressing.

Ears

1. Allow free drainage of bloody or clear fluid from internal ear.
2. Leave foreign bodies in place to be removed at the hospital.

    Request paramedic evaluation if indicated by significant physical findings as listed in Appendix 12.

SPECIAL CONSIDERATIONS

1. The face, scalp, and neck are richly supplied with arteries and veins, and wounds of these areas bleed heavily.
2. Suspect brain or neck injuries with traumatic injuries to the face.

3. Remove impaled objects from the cheek and pack with dressings to protect airway from bleeding.

Fractures, Dislocations, and Sprains

DESCRIPTION

Injuries to the structures of the musculoskeletal system can result in fractures, dislocations, and sprains. A *fracture* is a break, chip, crack, or splinter of any bone. These can be open or closed. A *dislocation* occurs when one end of a bone making up a joint is pulled out of place. *Sprains* are injuries in which ligaments, those structures connecting bone to bone, are torn or stretched. These injuries should be treated prior to transport to minimize further damage.

SIGNIFICANT PHYSICAL FINDINGS

1. Localized pain and tenderness
2. Swelling, discoloration
3. Deformity, deep lacerations, exposed bone fragments
4. Crepitus or grating sound produced by the fractured ends of bone rubbing together
5. Loss of function, limitation of motion, guarding
6. Loss of pulses distal to injury

SIGNIFICANT HISTORY

1. History of trauma
2. Mechanism of injury
3. Previous medical problems
4. Current medication

PATIENT CARE

1. Control serious bleeding and dress open wounds.
2. Check for the impairment of circulation and nerve function.
3. Check for finger or toe movement and slight hand or foot movement.

4. *Fractures with a pulse:* Attempt to return extremity to anatomical position until resistance or pain is encountered; splint and elevate extremity.
5. *Fractures without a pulse:* Attempt to return extremity to anatomical position until pulse returns or resistance or pain is encountered, and splint.
6. *Femur fractures:* Apply traction and splint.
7. Splint all dislocations as they lie *except* with loss of pulse. In that case, attempt to straighten into anatomical position until pulse returns or resistance or pain is encountered.
8. Support fracture site while splinting.
9. Consider use of medical antishock trousers for stabilization of femur and pelvic fractures.
10. Consider starting a large-bore IV.
11. Immobilize joint injuries in position found.
12. Immobilize the joint above and below the fracture or dislocation.
13. Pad splint to prevent pressure points.
14. Splint all fractures before moving the patient.
15. Check pulses before and after splinting and leave pulse points open for assessing arterial blood flow.
16. Elevate extremity after splinting. Place cold pack over site.
17. Monitor for signs of shock from possible internal bleeding.
18. Provide proper care for sprains.
    a. Place the joint at absolute rest in an elevated position.
    b. Pack the sprained area in ice to reduce swelling, control internal bleeding, and reduce pain.
    c. Apply a pillow or blanket splint, then transport.
19. Request paramedic evaluation if indicated by significant physical findings as listed in Appendix 12.

SPECIAL CONSIDERATIONS

1. Even when a dislocation is believed to have occurred, a combined injury of dislocation and fracture is possible. If unclear as to whether a dislocation or fracture, treat as a dislocation and splint as it lies unless there is loss of pulse.
2. Do not apply ice or cold packs directly to skin. Wrap cold pack in a cloth.

Femur Fractures

DESCRIPTION

Fractures to the midshaft of the femur are often associated with injuries to large blood vessels and nerves. Internal and/or external bleeding can be severe enough to cause shock. Care of femur fractures requires the application of traction and a splint to reduce pain and minimize blood loss.

SIGNIFICANT PHYSICAL FINDINGS

1. Intense pain and swelling
2. Deformity, angulation, or rotation of the injured leg
3. Injured leg appears shorter
4. Open wound and bleeding
5. Inability to move toes below site of injury
6. Loss of a pulse below injury

SIGNIFICANT HISTORY

1. Mechanism of injury
2. Significant medical problems, current medications
3. Known allergies

PATIENT CARE

1. Immobilize on a backboard.
2. Apply traction by one of the following methods:
   a. Medical antishock trousers with a Sager splint if available (considered to be the best method for treating femur fractures). Inflate until firm unless patient in shock, requiring full inflation.
   b. Traction splint or Thomas half-ring if MAST unavailable.
   c. Medical antishock trousers alone if only equipment or if multiple patients involved.
3. Treat for shock. If SBP below 90 and pulse above 110, or SBP below 80 regardless of pulse, apply and inflate antishock trousers if available.
4. Consider starting IV with a large-bore needle.

> 5. Keep checking pulse distal to injury.
> 6. Request paramedic evaluation if indicated by significant physical findings as listed in Appendix 12.

SPECIAL CONSIDERATION

Save any pieces of bone and transport with the patient as an amputated part.

Hip Injuries (High Femur) in the Elderly

DESCRIPTION

Dislocation versus fracture to the head of the femur is often difficult to distinguish. Hip dislocation is when the head of the femur slips out of the hip socket. A hip fracture is a break in the upper level of the femur or a fracture of the socket. Hip fractures are common among elderly patients, who often fall while standing or walking. Fractures of the hip in elderly patients are less often associated with significant bleeding and shock.

SIGNIFICANT PHYSICAL FINDINGS

1. Localized intense pain, sometimes pain in the knee
2. Discoloration of surrounding tissue
3. Swelling
4. Inability to move limb or flex the foot while lying on back
5. Foot on injured side turns outward, entire limb rotates inward or outward
6. Injured leg appears shorter
7. Signs of shock: altered consciousness; rapid, weak pulse; cool, clammy skin; low blood pressure; paleness

SIGNIFICANT HISTORY

1. Mechanism and force of injury
2. Age of patient
3. Previous fractures and hospitalizations
4. Current medical problems and medications

> **PATIENT CARE**
>
> 1. Utilize clamshell carrier to move patient to long backboard.
> 2. Immobilize on a backboard per guidelines avoiding any pressure over fracture site.
> 3. Treat for shock. If SBP below 90 and pulse rate above 110 or a SBP below 80 regardless of pulse, apply and inflate antishock trousers if available.
> 4. Apply ECG monitor.
> 5. Consider starting an IV.
> 6. Continue to reevaluate pulse distal to injury.
> 7. Request paramedic evaluation if indicated by significant physical findings as listed in Appendix 12.

Hip Injuries (High Femur) in the Young

DESCRIPTION

Dislocation versus fracture of the head of the femur is often difficult to distinguish. Hip dislocation is when the head of the femur slips out of the hip socket. A hip fracture is a break in the upper level of the femur or a fracture of the socket. Internal bleeding and shock are serious complications of traumatic hip fractures in the young.

SIGNIFICANT PHYSICAL FINDINGS

1. Localized intense pain, sometimes pain in the knee
2. Discoloration of surrounding tissue
3. Swelling
4. Inability to move limb or flex the foot while lying on back
5. Foot on injured side turns outward, or entire limb rotates inward or outward
6. Injured leg appears shorter
7. Signs of shock: altered level of consciousness; rapid, weak pulse; cool, clammy skin; low blood pressure; paleness
8. Absent pulse distal to injury

SIGNIFICANT HISTORY

1. Mechanism and force of injury
2. Age of patient
3. Previous fractures and hospitalizations
4. Current medical problems and medications

PATIENT CARE

1. Administer oxygen.
2. Secure antishock trousers (if available) to long backboard.
3. Utilize clamshell carrier to move patient to long backboard.
4. Apply and inflate MAST until firm unless patient in shock requiring full inflation. Immobilize on backboard.
5. Treat for shock. If SBP below 90 and pulse rate above 110 or a SBP below 80 regardless of pulse, apply and inflate antishock trousers if available.
6. Consider starting an IV with a large-bore needle.
7. Continue to monitor pulse distal to injury.
8. Request paramedic evaluation if indicated by significant physical findings as listed in Appendix 12.

Pelvic Injuries

DESCRIPTION

Pelvic fractures usually result from a direct blow or from a squeeze on the hips. Trauma to the pelvis can cause injuries to the organs of the lower abdomen, which include the bladder, rectum, and internal female sex organs. Injury to these organs can lead to serious internal bleeding and shock. Assume spinal injury in such patients.

SIGNIFICANT PHYSICAL FINDINGS

1. Severe pain at fracture site
2. Pain when pressure is applied to pelvis or pubic bone
   a. Compression of the iliac crests
      (1) Laterally
      (2) Anteriorly
   b. Compression of the pubic symphysis, anteriorly

3. Inability to lift legs
4. Signs of shock: altered consciousness; rapid, weak pulse; cool, clammy skin; low blood pressure; paleness

SIGNIFICANT HISTORY

1. Mechanism and force of injury
2. Current medical problems and medications

PATIENT CARE

1. Assess for life-threatening injuries and treat first.
2. Administer oxygen.
3. Move the patient as little as possible. Never lift patient without supporting pelvis.
4. Place antishock trousers (MAST) if available on backboard before positioning patient.
5. Lift patient to backboard using clamshell stretcher.
6. Assess femoral pulses for equalness.
7. Apply and inflate MAST until firm. If patient in shock, inflate until pop-off valves release.
8. If MAST unavailable, pad both sides of pelvis with rolled blankets and place folded blanket between patient's legs and bind them together with wide cravats.
9. Consider starting an IV with a large-bore needle.
10. Continue to reevaluate pulses distal to injury site.
11. Monitor vital signs closely for signs of shock.
12. Paramedic evaluation required; if paramedics unavailable, transport immediately.

SPECIAL CONSIDERATIONS

1. Any force strong enough to fracture the pelvis can also cause injury to the spine.
2. If in doubt as to whether fracture is to pelvis or head of femur, use the medical antishock trousers rather than a traction splint.
3. Use of MAST is not appropriate if there is evidence of internal rotation of a lower extremity, suggesting posterior dislocation of the hip.

Spinal Cord Injuries

DESCRIPTION

Forty-three percent of all spinal cord injuries occur in motor vehicle accidents. Damage to the spinal cord can result in partial or complete paralysis or death. Proper management and handling are critical to the patient's survival. Any patient involved in a traumatic accident should be assessed and treated for possible spinal injury.

SIGNIFICANT PHYSICAL FINDINGS

1. Pain in the neck or spine
2. Tenderness upon palpation of area
3. Deformity such as abnormal bend or bony prominence
4. Cuts and bruises about the head, face, shoulder, abdomen
5. Paralysis
6. Loss of sensation or numbness
7. Painful movement if patient tries to move
8. Priapism (male erection)
9. Rapid pulse
10. Low blood pressure
11. Dry, warm skin
12. No findings—significant when considering mechanism of injury

SIGNIFICANT HISTORY

1. Mechanism of injury; forceful trauma above the level of the femurs
2. Current medical problems and medications

PATIENT CARE

1. Administer oxygen.
2. Immobilize cervical spine with semirigid collar and manual support.
3. Position and immobilize on long backboard using cravats, Velcro straps, or belts.
   a. Secure forehead.

b. Crisscross across chest and under the arms.
   c. Loosely tie wrists together with Kling (preferred for comfort).
   d. Release traction of the head.
   e. Pad space around head.
   f. Pad small of back, behind knees, and between legs.
   g. Crisscross across pelvis but not over bladder.
   h. Place one strap straight across midthigh.
   i. Place one strap straight across midtibia.
   j. Place one strap straight across feet.
4. Treat for neurological shock by elevating foot of backboard or use of MAST if SBP below 90 and pulse above 110, or SBP below 80 regardless of pulse.
5. Repeat motor and sensory neurological check after immobilizing.
6. Monitor vital signs frequently during transport.
7. Consider applying ECG monitor.
8. Consider starting an IV with large-bore needle.
9. Paramedic evaluation required; if paramedics unavailable, transport immediately.

SPECIAL CONSIDERATIONS

1. Be prepared to tip backboard on its side if patient begins to vomit, and have suction available.
2. If patient has sustained high cord injury, breathing is diaphragmatic. If using MAST, monitor respirations closely for deterioration.
3. If shock is severe, look for evidence of internal bleeding.
4. Mechanism of injury, in absence of significant physical findings, should be an indication for spinal immobilization.
5. If an extrication device or shortboard was used during extrication, after securing patient to the long backboard, release as many shortboard chest straps as needed to allow comfortable chest expansion.
6. Continuously reevaluate the patient's status. Do not spend an excessive amount of time physically immobilizing critical patients needing resuscitation.

Throat Injuries

DESCRIPTION

In traumatic accidents, the throat is usually injured by a blunt or crushing blow. Impact with a steering wheel or dashboard, hanging by attempted suicide, or contact with a stretched wire or rope are common causes of throat injuries. Severe bleeding from a lacerated artery, air embolism from a torn vein, airway obstruction from a crushed larynx or trachea, or spinal cord damage are serious complications of throat injuries.

SIGNIFICANT PHYSICAL FINDINGS

1. Altered or loss of voice
2. Noisy breathing
3. Respiratory difficulty
4. Deformity, contusions, or depressions in the neck
5. Swelling and discoloration of the neck, face, or chest
6. Bright red, spurting blood, indicating arterial bleed; can be coughing up blood
7. Profuse, steady flow of dark red blood, indicating venous bleeding

SIGNIFICANT HISTORY

1. Mechanism of injury, penetrating or blunt trauma
2. Current medical problems and medications

PATIENT CARE

1. Assist respirations as necessary.
2. Administer high flow (10 to 15 LPM) of oxygen by mask.
3. Control arterial bleeding.
   a. Apply direct pressure with bulky dressing. Continue to add dressings.
   b. Avoid pressure over the airway or on both sides of the neck.

c. Apply pressure to carotid pressure point if necessary. Do not apply pressure on both carotid arteries at the same time.
4. Control venous bleeding and prevent air embolism.
   a. Apply direct pressure with bulky dressing.
   b. Apply pressure above and below point of bleeding if not immediately controlled by direct pressure.
   c. Apply occlusive dressing or saran wrap and tape all edges once bleeding is controlled.
5. Assess for spinal injuries and immobilize as necessary.
6. Monitor airway and vital signs.
7. Request paramedic evaluation if indicated by significant physical findings as listed in Appendix 12.

Appendices

APPENDIX 1: BAG-VALVE-MASK (FATS) TECHNIQUE

1. Choose correct size mask for the patient. Place apex or top of the triangular mask over the bridge of the nose (between the eyebrows). The base of the mask should rest between the patient's lower lip and the prominence of the chin.
2. To hold mask firmly in position:
   a. Place heel of hand on top of mask or valve.
   b. The fingers and thumb should extend straight forward.
   c. Lower hand to grasp jaw with middle two or three fingers.
3. Using head tilt, chin-lift open the airway by sitting back on the heels, tilting the head while lifting the chin with the hand on the mask or valve.
4. Squeeze knees together to keep patient's head hyperextended. This helps to stabilize the neck, also to take pressure off the hand holding the mask in place so that the hand can concentrate on maintaining the seal.
5. Make sure pressure is applied at the same angle as the facepiece to the face, to get even distribution of pressure and a proper seal.
6. With your other hand, squeeze the bag against your thigh once every 5 seconds. (Squeezing should cause the patient's chest to rise.)
7. Release pressure on the bag and let the patient passively exhale and the bag refill from the atmosphere or oxygen source.

APPENDIX 2: COMMUNITY RESOURCES

Agency	Reasons to Call
Alcohol and drug 24-hour	Resource for persons seeking help
Communicable disease control	Immunization information, exposure to infectious diseases
County sheriff's department	Follow-up of criminal cases, report suspicions of criminal activity
Domestic violence hotline	
Mental health clinic	Mentally ill patients not serious enough to hospitalize, but in need of professional counseling
Mental health professionals (available 24 hours)	Resource agency for concerned parents, relatives, etc.
Poison control center	Ingestion of substances
Childrens medical center	
Rape relief	Support for rape victims
Sexual assault center	
SIDS (sudden infant death syndrome)	Support and counseling for parents of SIDS victims
SIDS referral agency	
Suicide crisis line	
Victim services	Counseling and legal advice to victims of violent crime

APPENDIX 3: CONVERSION TABLES

Temperature Equivalents (°F)

98° (rectal) = 97° (oral) = 97° (forehead) = 96° (axillary)
99° (rectal) = 98° (oral) = 98° (forehead) = 97° (axillary)
100° (rectal) = 99° (oral) = 99° (forehead) = 98° (axillary)

Rule of thumb: rectal temperature 1° higher than an oral or forehead temperature; 2° higher than an axillary temperature

Liquid Measurements

1 tsp	=	5 cc = $\frac{1}{6}$ oz
1 tbsp	=	15 cc = $\frac{1}{2}$ oz
2 tbsp	=	30 cc = 1 oz
1 cup	=	240 cc = 8 oz
1 pint	=	500 cc = 16 oz
1 quart	=	1000 cc = 32 oz

Temperature

Celsius	
$(C° \times 9/5) + 32 = F°$	$(F° - 32) \times 5/9 = C°$
0	32
35.0	96.8
36.5	97.7
37.0	98.6
37.5	99.5

APPENDIX 3: CONVERSION TABLES (*Continued*)

Linear measurements	
1 millimeter (mm)	= 0.04 inch
1 centimeter (cm)	= 0.4 inch
2.5 centimeters	= 1 inch
1 meter	= 39.37 inches

Weight Equivalents	
1 oz =	30 grams
1 kg =	1000 grams
1 kg =	2.2 lb
1 lb =	0.45 kg

Temperature	
Celsius	
$(C° \times 9/5) + 32 = F°$	$(F° - 32) \times 5/9 = C°$
38.0	100.4
38.5	101.3
39.0	102.2
39.5	103.1
40.0	104.0
40.5	104.9
41.0	105.8
41.5	106.7
42.0	107.6

APPENDIX 4: DIABETIC COMA AND SHOCK FACT SHEET

Signs and Symptoms	Diabetic Coma (Ketoacidosis)	Insulin Shock (Low Blood Sugar)
Appearance	Extremely ill	Very weak
Skin	Red and dry	Pale
Mouth	Dry	Drooling
Thirst	Intense	Absent
Hunger	Absent	Intense
Respiratory	Exaggerated air hunger	Normal to shallow
Breath	Acetone	Normal
BP	Low	Normal
Pulse	Rapid	Normal or may be rapid
Mental state	Restless, merging into unconsciousness	Apathy, irritability
Tremor	Absent	Frequent
Improvement	Gradual, 6–12 hours	Immediate, within minutes of carbohydrate administration

Source: Reprinted from *Washington State Field Protocols.*

APPENDIX 5: DRUGS COMMONLY PRESCRIBED

Drug	Indications for Use
Acetaminophen	Fever, pain inflammation
Adapin	Depression
Aladactone	High blood pressure
Aldomet	High blood pressure
Alupent	Bronchospasms, asthma, COPD
Aminophylline	Bronchospasms, asthma, COPD
Amitriptyline	Depression
Antivert	Nausea and vomiting
Apresoline	High blood pressure
Asendin	Depression
Aspirin	Fever, pain, inflammation
Atarax	Anxiety, tension, sedation
Benadryl	Allergic reactions
Blocadren	Angina, high blood pressure
Bricanyl	Asthma, bronchospasms
Bronkosol	Asthma, coronary artery spasms, arrhythmias
Calan	Asthma, bronchospasms
Capoten	CHF, hypertension
Cardiozem	Angina, coronary artery spasm
Catapress	High blood pressure
Centrax	Anxiety
Cimetidine	Ulcers
Clinoril	Arthritis
Clonopin	Seizures
Corgard	Angina, hypertension
Coumadin	Blood thinner
Darvocet	Pain
Darvon	Pain
Depakene	Seizures
Diabinese	Diabetes
Diazepam	Anxiety, seizures
Digoxin	CHF, arrhythmias
Dilantin	Seizures
Dimetap	Allergic reactions
Diphenhydramine	Allergic reactions
Dipyridamole	Angina
Diuril	High blood pressure
Dyazide	High blood pressure
Dymelor	Diabetes
Elavil	Depression
Endep	Depression

APPENDIX 5: DRUGS COMMONLY PRESCRIBED (*Continued*)

Drug	Indications for Use
Enduron	CHF
Feldene	Pain, inflammation, arthritis
Furosemide	High blood pressure, CHF, edema
Gaviscon	Ulcers
Haldol	Psychosis; promotes sleep (sedation)
Heparin	Blood thinner
Hydralazine	High blood pressure
Hydrochlorothiazide	High blood pressure, CHF
Hydro-dyril	High blood pressure, CHF
Hygroton	High blood pressure, CHF
Ibuprofen	Inflammation, arthritis
Imipramine	Depression
Inderal	Angina, arrhythmias, high blood pressure
Indocin	Arthritis, inflammation
Isordil	Angina
Isuprel	Bronchospasms, asthma
Lanoxin	CHF, arrhythmias
Lasix	High blood pressure, edema, CHF
Librax	Ulcers, irritable bowel syndrome
Librium	Anxiety
Lithium	Manic-depression
Lopressor	High blood pressure
Maalox	Ulcers
Meclizine	Allergic reactions
Mellaril	Psychosis
Meprobamate	Anxiety, tension, sedation
Methadone	Drug addiction, pain, sedation
Miltown	Anxiety, tension, sedation
Minipress	High blood pressure
Moduretic	High blood pressure, CHF
Motrin	Arthritis, inflammation
Mylanta	Ulcers
Mysoline	Seizure
Nardil	Depression
Navane	Psychosis
Nifedipine	Angina, coronary artery spasm
Nitrobid, paste	Angina
Nitroglycerine	Angina
Norpace	Arrhythmias
Norpramin	Depression

APPENDIX 5: DRUGS COMMONLY PRESCRIBED
(Continued)

Drug	Indications for Use
Orinase	Diabetes
Parafon forte	Muscle cramps
Parnate	Depression
Pavabid	Angina, arrhythmias
Percodan	Pain
Percogesic	Pain
Phenobarbitol	Seizure, sedation
Presantine	Angina
Procain	Arrhythmias
Pronestol	Arrhythmias
Propranolol	Angina, arrhythmias, high blood pressure
Quinidex	Arrhythmias
Quinidine	Arrhythmias
Resperine	CHF, high blood pressure
Riopan	Ulcers
Serax	Anxiety, sedation
Sinequan	Depression
Stelazine	Psychosis
Tagamet	Ulcers
Tegretol	Seizures
Tenormin	Angina, high blood pressure
Theodur	Bronchospasms, asthma, COPD
Theophylline	Bronchospasms, asthma, COPD
Thiazide	High blood pressure
Thorazine	Psychosis
Timolol	Angina, high blood pressure
Tofranil	Depression, anxiety
Tolectin	Arthritis, inflammation
Tolinase	Diabetes
Tranxene	Anxiety
Triavil	Depression
Tylenol	Pain, fever, inflammation
Tylox	Pain
Valium	Anxiety, seizures
Ventolin	Bronchospasms, asthma, COPD
Verapamil	Angina, coronary artery spasm, arrhythmias
Vivactil	Depression
Warafin	Blood thinner
Zanax	Sedation
Zarontin	Seizures
Zyloprim	Gout

APPENDIX 6: MEDICAL ANTISHOCK TROUSERS (MAST) PROCEDURE

I. *Indications for Use*
   A. Multisystems trauma
   B. Shock
      1. Supine BP between 80 and 90 mmHg and pulse rate above 100 per minute
      2. Systolic BP below 80 mmHg regardless of pulse rate
   C. Nontraumatic patients in shock and bleeding without chest pain
   D. Splinting: femur and pelvic fractures
II. *Contraindicators for use*
   A. Absolute contraindicators for use
      1. Cardiogenic shock: nontraumatic chest pain
      2. Hypothermia: less than 90°F or 32°C
      3. Children under 12 years of age weighing less than 80 pounds
      4. Pulmonary edema
   B. Burns: second- or third-degree in area under trousers
      1. Dress and inflate all chambers if SBP below 80.
      2. Inflate legs only if burns are on abdomen when SBP is between 80 and 90, and pulse above 110.
   C. Abdominal inflation contraindicated (unless BP remains 80 after inflation of the legs)
      1. Pregnancy
      2. Evisceration of the abdomen
      3. Impaled objects in the abdomen
      4. Suspected tension pneumothorax
III. *Inflation Procedures*
   A. Inflate legs.
   B. Listen to lungs. If clear and unobstructed, proceed to abdominal section.
   C. Inflate abdominal chambers.
   D. Take and record vital signs after full inflation.
IV. *Special Consideration:* Any time the patient's condition warrants the inflation of the antishock trousers, a paramedic unit *must* be dispatched.

APPENDIX 7: MEDICAL INCIDENT REPORT FORM; SOAP REPORTING

	BLOOD PRESSURE	PULSE	RESP RATE	EYE OPENING	MOTOR RESPONSE	VERBAL RESPONSE	NAILBED (SECS)
INITIAL VITAL SIGNS [ ][ ][ ][ ] TIME	⚲ ⎵⎵⎵/⎵⎵⎵ ⚲ ⎵⎵⎵/⎵⎵⎵ ⚲ ⎵⎵⎵/⎵⎵⎵	⎵⎵⎵ ⎵⎵⎵ ⎵⎵⎵	⎵⎵⎵ /MIN EFFORT 1☐ Normal 0☐ Labored/absent	4☐ Spontaneously 3☐ To voice 2☐ To pain 1☐ No response	6☐ Obeys commands 5☐ Locates pain 4☐ W'draw from pain 3☐ Flexion to pain 2☐ Extension to pain 1☐ No response	5☐ Oriented 4☐ Confused 3☐ Inapproa. words 2☐ Incomprehensible 1☐ No response	2☐ 2 or less 1☐ More than 2 0☐ No response PUPILS 1☐ Equal 0☐ Not equal

FLOW CHART	TIME								
	Blood Pressure								
	Pulse Rate								
	Respiratory Rate								
	Consciousness								
	ECG Rhythm								
	IV fluids, liters:								
	Shock								

Medications Taken By Patient At Home:

Allergies:

Narrative (Subjective, Objective, Assessment, Plan):

S: Subjective information is what is told by patient or bystanders and includes: chief complaint (why did the patient call for help); mechanism of injury; medical history; relevant medical problems; recent illnesses or surgeries; allergies. Symptoms: what the patient is experiencing that cannot be observed.

O: Objective information is what was observed or found by the examiner upon arrival and during the patient exam.

A: Assessment is the examiner's idea of what is going on with the patient, and thus determines how the EMT will treat the patient.

P: Plan of treatment is what was done for the patient.

Any information posted to this form is based on observations made by EMS personnel, and is not necessarily a medical fact.

AGENCY COPY

FORM 911 4/87

APPENDIX 7: MEDICAL INCIDENT REPORT FORM; SOAP REPORTING (*Continued*)

	BLOOD PRESSURE	PULSE	RESP RATE	EYE OPENING	MOTOR RESPONSE	VERBAL RESPONSE	NAILBED (SECS)
INITIAL VITAL SIGNS [ ][ ][ ] TIME	○⌒ ⊔⊔⊔/⊔⊔⊔ ♀ ⊔⊔⊔/⊔⊔⊔ ♀ ⊔⊔⊔/⊔⊔⊔	⊔⊔⊔ ⊔⊔⊔ ⊔⊔⊔	⊔⊔ /MIN EFFORT 1☐ Normal 0☐ Labored/ absent	4☐ Spontaneously 3☐ To voice 2☐ To pain 1☐ No response	6☐ Obeys commands 5☐ Locates pain 4☐ W'draw from pain 3☐ Flexion to pain 2☐ Extension to pain 1☐ No response	5☐ Oriented 4☐ Confused 3☐ Inapproa. words 2☐ Incomprehensible 1☐ No response	2☐ 2 or less 1☐ More than 2 0☐ No response PUPILS 1☐ Equal 0☐ Not equal

	TIME								
FLOW CHART	Blood Pressure								
	Pulse Rate								
	Respiratory Rate								
	Consciousness								
	ECG Rhythm								
	IV fluids, liters:								
	Shock								

Medications Taken By Patient At Home: Allergies:

Narrative (Subjective, Objective, Assessment, Plan):

S: 21 yo ♂ with gunshot wound to chest. Said to have been struggling with assailant when gun went off at close range. C6 difficulty breathing. No current medical problems or known allergies.

O: On arrival, patient found lying supine. PD on scene applying pressure to open wound below right nipple. Single hole from small caliber gun, no exit wound. Vital signs: RR 20 and shallow; BP 80/50; pulse 130 and weak. Chest: breath sounds diminished on right side. Moderate amount of bleeding from wound. ABD: soft without masses.

A: Traumatic injury to chest with hypotension and respiratory distress.

P: (1) Pt. exam.
(2) Pressure dressing to wound.
(3) Oxygen at 10 LPM via non-rebreathing mask.
(4) Inflated legs of antishock trousers only.
(5) Medic 5 transported to HMC.

Any information posted to this form is based on observations made by EMS personnel, and is not necessarily a medical fact.

AGENCY COPY   FORM 911 4/87

APPENDIX 8: MEDICAL RADIO REPORT

The radio report is for providing concise information regarding patient status to the dispatch center, incoming paramedics, emergency department staff, and physicians.

A. *Identification*
   1. Responding department and unit number
   2. Patient: number, age, sex
B. *History*
   1. Mechanism of injury or chief complaint
   2. Important symptoms
   3. Past history only if pertinent: medications, similar problems in the past
C. *Objective Findings*
   1. Level of consciousness
   2. Vital signs
   3. Pertinent localized findings
D. *EMT Care:* What the EMT has done so far (e.g., oxygen at 2 LPM per cannula, applied and inflated MAST.)
E. *Estimated Time of Arrival to Hospital* (if transporting)
F. *Special Considerations*
   1. Outstanding objective findings may take precedence over history and need to be reported first.
   2. Radio reports broadcast potentially confidential and privileged information, so use discretion.
   3. The EMTs are requested to give a short report to the paramedics for the following:
      a. Patient status changes or differs from dispatcher report
      b. Any time the EMT requests assistance from paramedics
   4. If EMTs elect to transport patient, they would contact the receiving hospital regarding patient problem and condition, and estimated arrival time.
   5. Confirm dispatcher's report along with vital signs to incoming paramedics.

APPENDIX 9: METTAG USE FOR DISASTERS

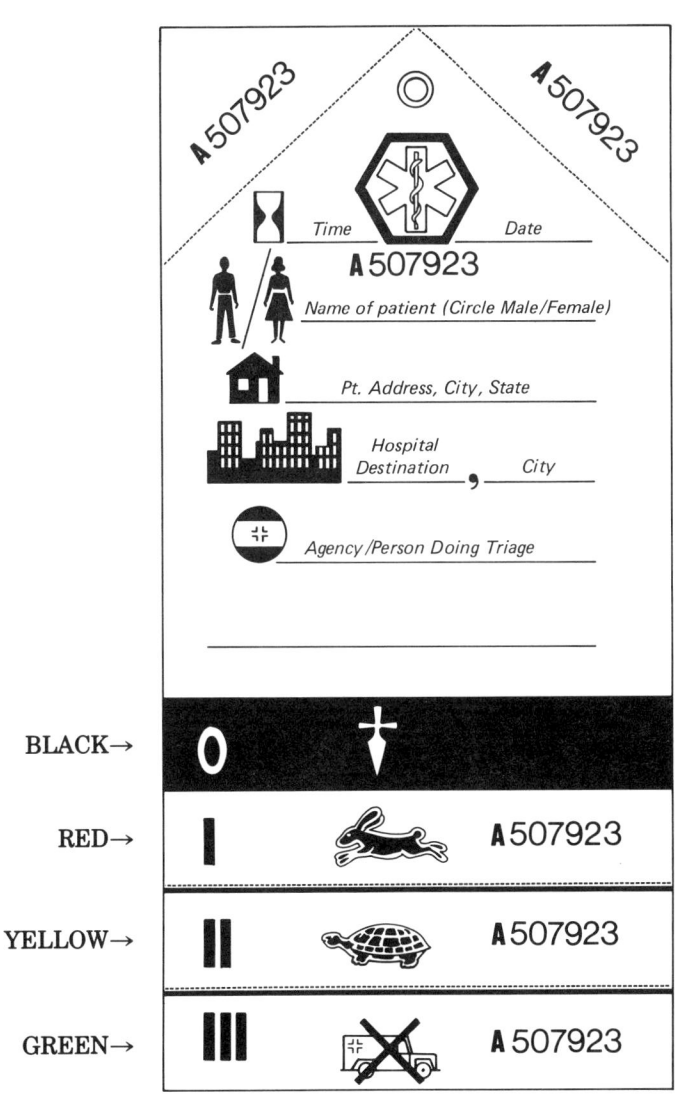

0: EXPECTED CATEGORY (BLACK)
Patients so critically injured only prolonged and complicated treatment is required, or patients who are dead.

I: PRIORITY I (RED)
Life-threatening condition requiring immediate, but limited, intervention to save life or limb.

II: PRIORITY II (YELLOW)
Stable patients who require basic field emergency care and hospitalization; transport can be delayed 30 minutes to 2 hours.

III: PRIORITY III (GREEN)
Ambulatory patients, minor or no treatment required; usually does not require in-patient treatment.

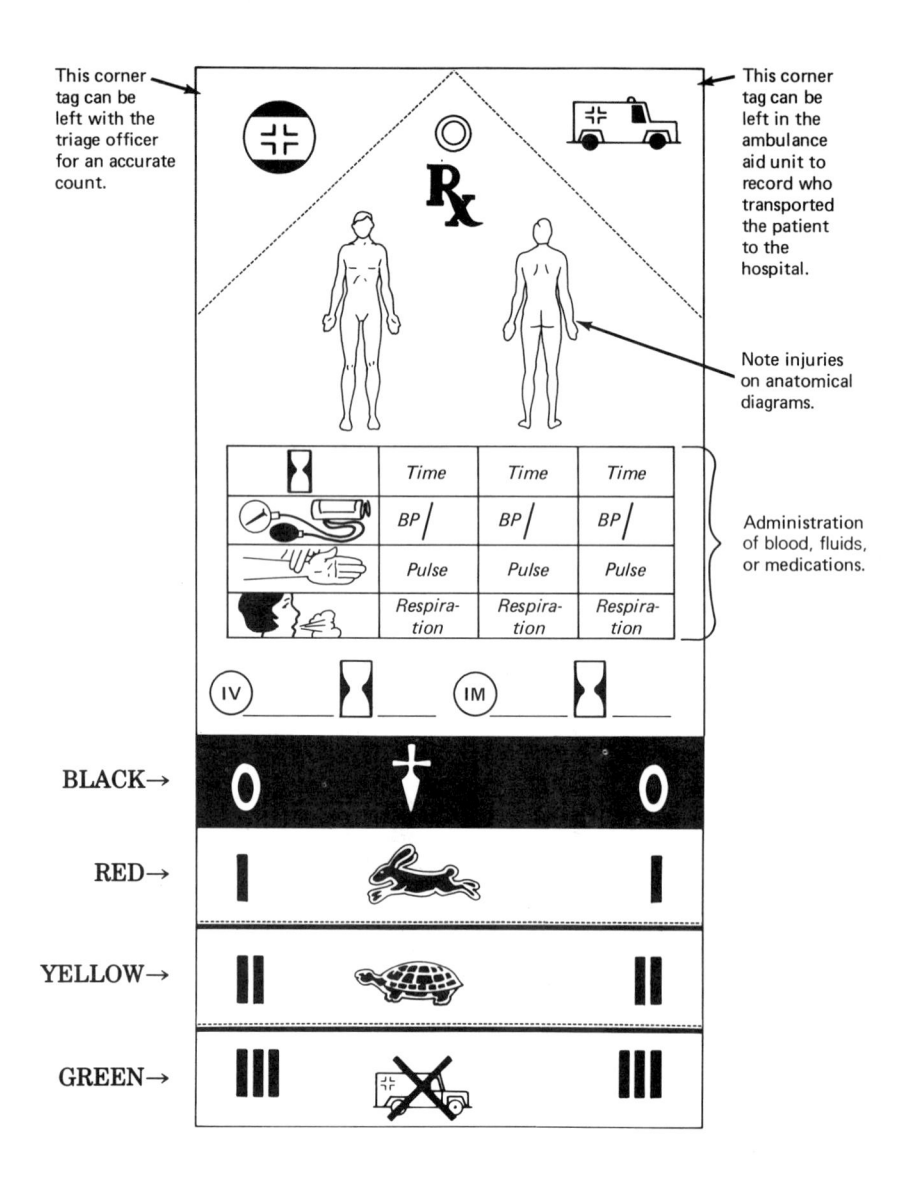

This corner tag can be left with the triage officer for an accurate count.

This corner tag can be left in the ambulance aid unit to record who transported the patient to the hospital.

Note injuries on anatomical diagrams.

Administration of blood, fluids, or medications.

BLACK→

RED→

YELLOW→

GREEN→

*Tear off all colored tabs BELOW determined priority and retain.

APPENDIX 10: TECHNIQUES OF HELMET REMOVAL[*]

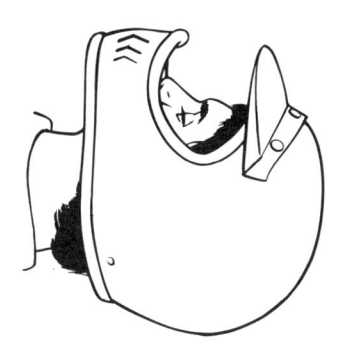

Although the repeal or modification of motorcycle helmet legislation in 37 states has significantly decreased helmet use (increasing motorcycle deaths), approximately 40 to 50 percent of motorcyclists wear helmets.[†] We believe that helmets do not cause neck injuries. As a matter of fact, a Kansas study showed that there was a slight decrease in the number of helmeted riders with neck injuries when compared to nonhelmeted riders. This difference is small, 52 percent as compared to 48 percent, and probably not statistically significant. It does indicate that there is no increased incidence of neck injuries with helmet use.

The aspect that can be confusing to the examining physician or prehospital-care technician is that the classical findings of face and head injuries, which indicate the need for cervical spine protection, may not exist. The helmet has protected the face and head from such injuries. Therefore, the helmet should be examined for abrasions or other signs of trauma. If they exist, the patient should be treated as if he had a cervical-spine fracture until lateral x-rays rule it out.

The physician, nurse, and prehospital-care personnel should understand the mechanisms of helmet removal in order to preserve an open airway, adequately stabilize the head to the short or long backboard, provide in-line fraction for moving a patient from automobile to gurney or from the gurney to an x-ray table, or to place Crutchfield or Gardner Wells tongs. Helmets are easily removed if one understands how they are built and how they conform to the shape of the head. If one does not understand this, helmet

---

[*] Reprinted from *Bulletin, American College of Surgeons,* October 1980.
[†] N. E. McSwain, Jr. and M. Lummis, Impact of repeal of motorcycle helmet law. *Surg. Gynecol. Obstet.* 151(2):215–224, 1980.

Types of helmets

Full face coverage — motorcycle, auto racer

Full face coverage — motocross

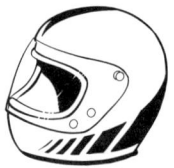

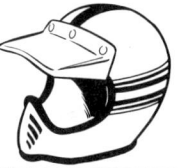

Helmet removal

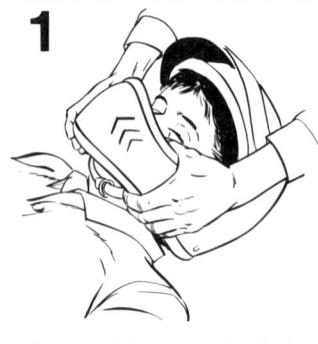

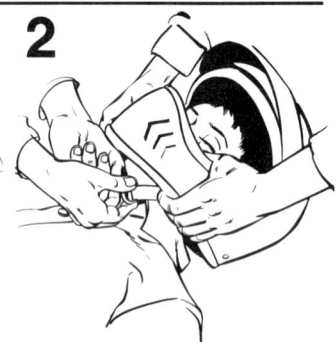

1

One rescuer applies inline traction by placing his or her hands on each side of the helmet with the fingers on the victim's mandible. This position prevents slippage if the strap is loose.

2

The rescuer cuts or loosens the strap at the D-rings while maintaining inline traction.

The varying sizes, shapes, and configurations of motorcycle helmets necessitate some understanding of their proper removal from victims of motorcycle accidents. The rescuer who removes a helmet improperly might inadvertently aggravate cervical spine injuries.

The Committee on Trauma believes that physicians who treat the injured should be aware of helmet removal techniques. A gradual increase in the use of helmets is anticipated because many organizations are urging voluntary wearing of helmets, and some states are reinstating their laws requiring the wearing of helmets.

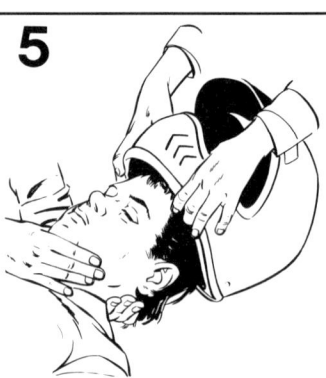

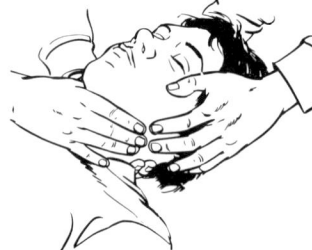

5

Throughout the removal process, the second rescuer maintains inline traction from below in order to prevent head tilt.

6

After the helmet has been removed, the rescuer at the top replaces his hands on either side of the victim's head with his palms over the ears.

American College of Surgeons Committee on Trauma
July 1980

Partial face coverage — motorcycle, auto racer

Light head protection — bicycle, kayak

Football

3

4

A second rescuer places one hand on the mandible at the angle, the thumb on one side, the long and index fingers on the other. With his other hand, he applies pressure from the occipital region. This maneuver transfers the inline traction responsibility to the second rescuer.

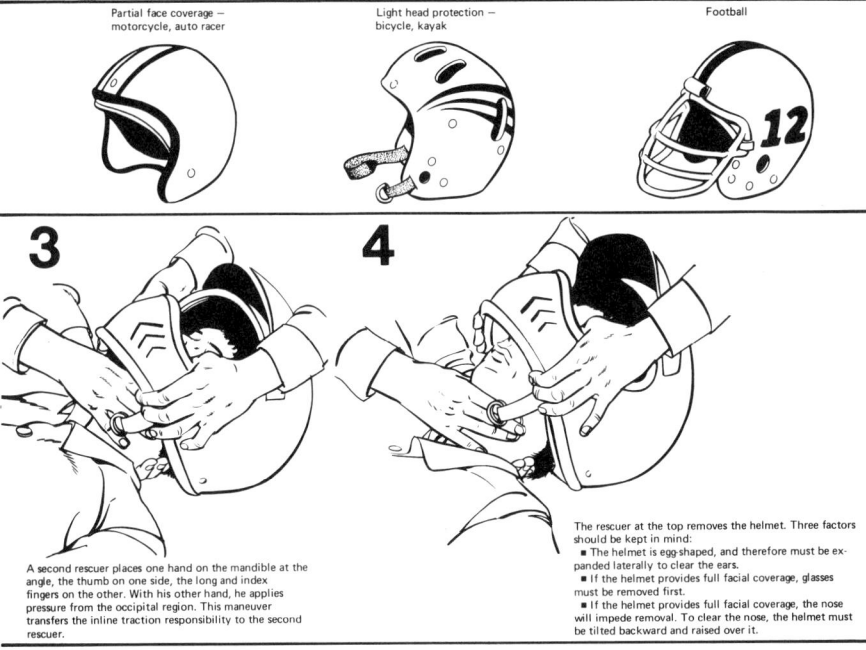

The rescuer at the top removes the helmet. Three factors should be kept in mind:
- The helmet is egg-shaped, and therefore must be expanded laterally to clear the ears.
- If the helmet provides full facial coverage, glasses must be removed first.
- If the helmet provides full facial coverage, the nose will impede removal. To clear the nose, the helmet must be tilted backward and raised over it.

7

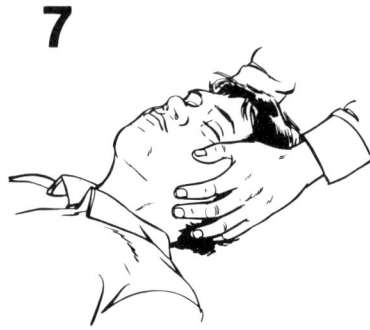

Inline traction is maintained from above until a backboard is in place.

Summary

The helmet must be maneuvered over the nose and ears while the head and neck are held rigid.
- Inline traction is applied from above.
- Inline traction is transferred below with pressure on the jaw and occiput.
- The helmet is removed.
  Inline traction is re-established from above.

removal can be very frustrating to the physician or other personnel dealing with the emergency patient. Inappropriate actions can damage the cervical cord when the overlying bony structure has been fractured.

For these reasons the Committee on Trauma has developed the accompanying helmet poster on pages 144 and 145.

Norman E. McSwain, Jr., MD, FACS
for the Committee on Trauma

APPENDIX 11: OXYGEN ADMINISTRATION

Device	Liters per Minute	Percent	Indications for use
Nasal cannula	2–6	25–40	Usually well tolerated; flow rate higher than 6 LPM is drying to the mucous membranes and uncomfortable for the patient; cannot accurately control oxygen concentration
Simple face mask	6–10	35–60	Preferred on trauma patients
Partial rebreathing mask	6–10	35–60	Flow rate should not be less than 6 LPM to maintain adequate airflow through the bag
Nonrebreathing mask	8–15	80–95	Preferred in the field because of the high oxygen concentrations that can be delivered; multiple injuries, shock; poorly tolerated by patients who complain of feelings of suffocation
Venturi Mask	The four adapter settings:		The mask of choice for patients with COPD and CO_2 retention; more accurate control of oxygen concentrations with adapter
	4	24	
	4	28	
	8	35	
	8	40	
Bag-valve-mask with oxygen reservoir	15	90	Cardiac arrest

APPENDIX 12: PARAMEDIC REQUEST: WHEN TO CALL FOR ADVANCED HELP

GENERAL APPEARANCE

Deciding when to call for advanced life support is not always obvious. EMTs who have treated many patients often are able to look at a patient and know that the patient is very sick just by their general appearance, even though vital signs and physical findings are normal. Follow your instincts and experience; if the patient looks ill, and you have paramedics available, call for assistance.

MECHANISM OF INJURY

Traumatic accidents commonly result in multiple injuries. Injuries to the head, chest, abdomen, neck/spine, or pelvis carry a high risk of serious complications that can be life threatening. Complications may develop rapidly or slowly over several hours. When considering the potential for serious injury, consider the following:

Type of accident: motorcycle, automobile, diving, fall, pedestrian, motor vehicle, bicycle

Force: speed of vehicle, head-on collisions

Impact: seat belts, impact with stationary objects, thrown from vehicle

SIGNIFICANT PHYSICAL FINDINGS

The presence of any one of the signs and symptoms listed below should alert the EMT to the potential seriousness of an injury or illness and the *need* to involve the paramedics:

Unconscious/unresponsive
Changing level of consciousness
Disorientation, confusion, combativeness, agitation
Labored, noisy, or abnormal respirations
Rapid respirations: above 30 per minute; inability to speak in full sentences
Slow respirations: below 8 per minute
Weak, irregular pulse
Low blood pressure: below 90 mmHg systolic
High blood pressure: above 180 mmHg systolic, and/or diastolic above 120 mmHg
Postural changes in vital signs
   Increase in pulse rate of greater than 20 per minute
   Decrease in systolic BP or diastolic BP of greater than 20 mmHg
   Dizziness, fainting, lightheadedness while standing
Abnormal speech, loss of voice with trauma
Paralysis
Vomiting blood/passing bloody or tarry stools

SPECIAL CONDITIONS

Specific injuries, illnesses, and mechanisms of injury that generally require a paramedic response:

Anaphylaxis
Aneurysms
Arrest: cardiac and respiratory
Burns
    Facial
    Second- or third-degree
    Respiratory involvement
    Electrical burns or shock
Chest injuries
Chest pain
Childbirth emergencies and imminent delivery
Coma, unconsciousness
Congestive heart failure
Convulsions (*see* Seizures)
Croup
Decompression sickness (the bends)
Dehydration and hypovolemia in children
Delirium tremens
Drug overdose
Ectopic pregnancy
Epiglottitis
Exposure to hazardous materials
Head injuries/or trauma sustained by the head
Heat stroke
Hypertensive emergencies
Hypothermia
Insulin shock/hypoglycemia
MAST use
Near-drowning
Pelvic fractures
Penetrating trauma (gunshot, stabbing)
Pneumothorax
Pulmonary edema

Respiratory distress
Seizures
  Status
  Pregnancy
  Drug-related
  First-time
Shock
Spinal Cord Injuries
Stroke associated with:
  History of cardiac disease
  Respiratory distress
  Unconsciousness

THE SHORT REPORT

If significant physical findings indicate the need for paramedic evaluation, this information should be relayed by radio, allowing paramedics to determine whether they should proceed to the scene.

APPENDIX 13: POSTURAL BLOOD PRESSURE AND HEART RATE

DESCRIPTION

Postural blood pressure and heart rate are measurements of changes in the systolic and diastolic blood pressure and the heart rate when a patient changes from a lying to a standing position. Blood pressure that is normal while lying down may fall drastically when the patient either sits or stands up. This is similar to what occurs when one stands quickly after resting and feels dizzy. Normally, the body rapidly adjusts to the change in position. For someone seriously ill, however, the body is unable to adjust, the blood pressure drops, and the pulse rate increases. The patient may even faint.

CAUSES

A fall in the postural blood pressure plus an increase in the pulse rate most often indicates loss of intravascular fluid, from either hemorrhage or dehydration. Causes include internal bleeding, excessive dehydration from vomiting and diarrhea, diabetes and hyperglycemia, and pneumonia.

INDICATIONS

Indications for checking postural blood pressure and heart rate include:

1. Patient complains of lightheadedness or dizziness.
2. Patient complains of generalized weakness without apparent reason.
3. Patient appears stable but has nonspecific complaints of illness.
4. Patient has fainted (syncopal episode) for unknown reasons.
5. Patient complains of nausea, vomiting, diarrhea.

PROCEDURE

1. Obtain both blood pressure and heart rate after the patient has been in a supine position for at least 2 minutes.
2. Have the patient move to a standing position for 1 minute, if possible. Observe the patient for dizziness or lightheadedness. If the patient cannot tolerate the standing position, record the blood pressure and heart rate in the sitting position. When necessary, permit the patient to return to a sitting or lying position.
3. After 1 minute in the standing position (sitting if necessary) repeat the blood pressure and heart rate. Have the patient resume a recumbent position.

INTERPRETATION

1. *Positive:* 20/20/20
   A decrease of 20 mmHg in the systolic blood pressure
   or
   A decrease of 20 mmHg in the diastolic blood pressure
   or
   An increase in the pulse rate of 20 per minute
2. *Positive:* Fainting while standing, or dizziness or lightheadedness while standing that requires the patient to lie down

SPECIAL CONSIDERATIONS

1. The purpose of measuring the postural blood pressure and heart rate is to detect *subtle* hypovolemia. In this respect:
   a. Changes in heart rate are more sensitive than changes in blood pressure.
   b. Standing is more sensitive than sitting.

2. Positive changes in the adult indicate that *at least* 1000 cc of intravascular volume has been lost.

APPENDIX 14: RESTRAINTS FOR AGGRESSIVE OR VIOLENT PATIENTS

The use of physical restraints for patients who pose a threat to themselves or others is indicated only as the last resort. If restraints are used, care must be taken to protect the patient from possible injury.

1. Request police assistance.
2. A minimum of four people, one per extremity, must be available to assist.
3. Each member is assigned a specific limb.
4. On command from the team leader, the patient's limbs and head are immobilized in one coordinated effort.
5. Each extremity is restrained in the following manner (padded leather restraints are recommended):
    a. Secure one arm above the head and the other arm at waist level.
    b. Secure the head.
    c. Secure the feet.
6. Never leave alone a patient in restraints.
7. In the event of vomiting, carefully monitor the patient to prevent aspiration.

APPENDIX 15: VITAL SIGNS

Age	Pulse	Respirations	Blood Pressure	
			Average Systolic	Average Diastolic
Newborn (1–28 days)	110–150	60	80	46
3 months	110–140	40	89	60
6–12 months	100–140	30	89	60
1 year	100–140	25	89	60
2 years	90–100	20	98	64
3–5 years	80–100	20	100	70
10 years	70–100	15	114	60
Adolescent	70–100	12	118	60
Adult	60–100	12	120	70

APPENDIX 16: EMERGENCY INTRAVENOUS FLUID THERAPY

This EMT skill requires a special training program and regular practice to perform efficiently. The equipment used and types of fluid preferred for each emergency vary widely throughout the medical community. These guidelines recommend when to consider IV fluid therapy for each emergency patient. Refer to the textbook *Emergency Care,* Fourth Edition, (Grant, Murray, Bergeron, 1986), pp. 603–611, for specifics of this skill.

It is recommended that emergency initiation of prehospital IVs follow this rule: Two attempts or two minutes are allowed for IV initiation to avoid undue delay in patient transport. All other attempts are performed enroute.

APPENDIX 17: COMMUNICABLE DISEASE PREVENTION

It is recommended that emergency medical personnel take the following precautions against the transmission of communicable diseases. Each recommendation is explained in detail in the following sections.

1. Wear appropriate protective gear when there is potential contact with blood, body fluids, or feces.
2. Handle needles and sharps with extreme caution.
3. Use resuscitation devices to ventilate patients.
4. Wash thoroughly before and after patient care, especially after contact with blood or body fluids.
5. Clean and disinfect EMS vehicles and equipment appropriately.
6. Dispose of all wastes safely.
7. Report suspected exposures to designated supervisor.

Immunizations

To fight illness, it is important to maintain good health, use effective protective measures, and receive appropriate immunizations. The following immunizations are currently recommended.

1. Hepatitis B
2. Influenza
3. Measles-mumps-rubella (MMR)
4. Tetanus-diptheria (Td)
5. Tuberculosis skin test

Routine vaccination is *not* recommended for tuberculosis or typhoid, nor is routine immune globulin prophylaxis for hepatitis A.

Signs and Symptoms of Communicable Disease

Good preventive techniques should be followed routinely—many illnesses are communicable before symptoms appear, and others do not have obvious symptoms. Good practice is to use protective measures when treating all patients, and to treat all patients with respect. It is appropriate to explain to patients that measures such as gloves are for the patient's protection as well as the care provider's.

Signs and symptoms include, *but are not limited to,* those listed below. Remember that symptoms may not always indicate communicable disease, and that communicable diseases may not always present symptoms. Be conservative and practice good patient care and disease control at all times.

1. Diarrhea
2. Rash and/or fever of unknown origin
3. Draining wounds
4. Jaundice
5. Dialysis
6. Vomiting
7. Difficulty breathing with fever
8. Fever alone
9. Sore throat
10. Lymphadenopathy (swollen lymph nodes)
11. Severe headache
12. Stiff neck with fever

13. Red eyes
14. Cough

Protective Gear

Wear appropriate protective gear when potential contact with blood, body secretions, and tissue specimens. As a safeguard, all blood, body secretions, and tissue specimens should be treated as if they were contaminated. It is recommended that emergency medical personnel wear protective disposable gloves on a routine basis when skin contact with such materials is likely, both during treatment and when cleaning up, especially if personnel have open cuts or abrasions. Safety glasses are advisable when spattering is likely. Routine use of disposable masks is unnecessary—unless mouth-to-mouth is performed, the probability of disease transmission through oral/respiratory secretions is low. If EMS providers are aware that the patient has a communicable disease that is spread through oral or respiratory secretions (e.g., meningitis or tuberculosis), masking the patient is preferable. Disposable gowns or properly laundered cloth gowns can help protect clothing when blood is spattering or is present in large quantities; they are not necessary for routine use.

Needles and Sharps

Handle needles and sharps with extreme caution. Used needles can transmit bloodborne diseases such as hepatitis B, AIDS, and syphilis. Needles, scalpel blades, and other sharp objects should be treated as potentially infective once they have been used. Place disposable items into puncture-resistant sharps containers, located as close as possible to the area of use. Do not recap, bend, or purposefully break needles. While on a call, it may be more convenient to place used needles in a small block of Styrofoam for later disposal in a sharps container. Be sure that the Styrofoam is large enough to hold the longest needle used.

Resuscitation Technique

Use resuscitation devices to ventilate patients. Minimize mouth-to-mouth resuscitation by using mouthpieces, resuscitation bags, or other ventilation devices. Using a ventilation device instead of mouth-to-mouth will help protect against diseases spread by oral secretions. These diseases include chickenpox, measles, rubella, meningitis, pertussis, hepatitis B, tuberculosis, and cold and flu. There is no evidence that AIDS is spread by contact with saliva.

If a ventilation device is not available, wash hands and face thoroughly with soap and water and change any soiled clothing after performing mouth-to-mouth resuscitation. Clean and disinfect ventilation devices after each use.

Handwashing

Wash thoroughly before and after patient care, especially after contact with blood or body secretions. Change clothing soiled with blood or body secretions.

WHEN TO WASH

In the absence of a true emergency, *always* wash hands before and after caring for patients (even if you have worn gloves!) *and especially:*

1. Before performing invasive procedures
2. Before caring for newborns and patients who are severely immunocompromised
3. Before and after touching wounds
4. After contact with mucous membranes, blood or body fluids, secretions, or excretions (wash all exposed parts)
5. After touching objects that are likely to be contaminated
6. After taking care of a patient with a known infection

When in doubt, wash!

TECHNIQUE

General Guidelines

1. When handwashing is indicated, wash immediately after treating patient. Do not smoke, eat, or touch people or objects unnecessarily until hands have been washed.

2. Wash with an approved soap and, whenever possible, with water. It is recommended that aid cars and medic units carry water jugs with spigots for washing when running water is unavailable. If no water is available, use waterless cleansers, as indicated below.
3. Because many handwashing agents are drying to the skin, after washing use hand lotion to prevent chapping and dermatitis.

When Water Is Available

1. Remove disposable gloves slowly and carefully by rolling inside out. Dispose in garbage container lined with plastic bag.
2. Remove rings (and watch, if necessary) and clean them as you wash and disinfect hands.
3. Use an appropriate handwashing agent. The Centers for Disease Control states that for routine activities, plain soap and water appear to be sufficient to wash off most microorganisms. Antimicrobial or viricidal products actually kill or inhibit the growth of disease-causing microorganisms and are indicated before handling newborns and immunocompromised patients, or for an extra margin of safety for routine use. Disposable pump dispensers are highly recommended.
4. Rub all surfaces of lathered hands *vigorously* for *at least* 15 seconds. Use a scrub brush if available. Friction helps remove microorganisms.
5. Rinse thoroughly under a stream of water.
6. Turn off water with paper towel.
7. Dry hands with paper towel.
8. Do not reexpose hands by touching contaminated surfaces (see equipment cleaning guidelines). Pay special attention to radio equipment, vehicle door handles, spotlight handles, flashlights, box handles, pens and pencils, and medical equipment.

When Water Is Not Available

1. Remove disposable gloves slowly and carefully, by rolling inside out. Dispose in garbage container lined with plastic bag.

2. Remove rings and watch, and if they have been exposed, clean them as you wash your hands.
3. Use a product that can be used without water (e.g., Hibistat, Alcare, Cal-stat).
4. Rub hands together *vigorously* for at least 15 seconds.
5. Wash with appropriate soap and water as soon as possible.

Cleaning Vehicles and Equipment

Clean and disinfect EMS vehicles and equipment appropriately. Some viruses and microorganisms can stay alive outside the body for weeks, so it is important to remove them from vehicle and equipment surfaces. Document cleaning by recording date and times items are cleaned.

BACKGROUND

Cleaning is the physical removal of organic material or soil from objects—usually with water and soap or detergent.

Disinfection is the killing of infectious agents outside the body by pasteurization or chemical means.

Sterilization is the destruction of all forms of microbial life by steam under pressure, liquid or gaseous chemicals, or dry heat.

Equipment should be cleaned, disinfected, or sterilized, depending on its use. The Centers for Disease Control divides equipment into three categories:

I. *Critical items:* instruments or objects that are introduced directly into the bloodstream or into other normally sterile areas of the body. Examples are:
   Surgical instruments
   Cardiac catheters
   Implants
   Critical items must be sterilized.

II. *Semicritical items:* items that touch intact mucous membranes and have an intermediate risk of causing infection. Examples are:

Respiratory therapy equipment
Manikins

Semicritical items should be disinfected.

III. *Noncritical items:* items that do not ordinarily touch the patient or touch only intact skin. Examples are:
Blood pressure cuffs
Defibrillator
Stretcher
Walls and floor of vehicle

Cleaning alone is ordinarily sufficient for noncritical items, *except* when items have been exposed to known infectious materials or blood and body fluids. *Disinfect when exposure is known or likely.*

Sterilize	Disinfect	Clean
Category I:	*Category II:*	*Category III:*[a]
Surgical instruments	Bag mask	Air splints
Trach kits	Intubation equipment[b]	Backboards
	Portable suction[b]	C-collars
	Vehicle suction[b]	KED devices
	Vehicle work areas	Defibrillator MAST
	Blood spills	pants
	Catheter tips[b]	O$_2$ bottle
		Penrose tubing
		Splints and straps
		Stethoscope
		Stretcher and straps
		Vacuum splint/pump
		Vehicle walls and floor

[a] Category III items that have been exposed to blood or body fluids should be disinfected.
[b] Use high-level disinfection for parts exposed to mucous membranes.

METHODS

Cleaning: Use EPA-registered hospital-grade disinfectant-detergent or soap, depending on likelihood of contact with mucous membranes. Follow manufacturer's instructions, *scrub vigorously,* and rinse. Allow items to dry thoroughly.
High-level disinfection: Use hospital facilities or EPA-regis-

tered glutaraldehyde (e.g., Wavicide-01) product. Wear gloves, clean and rinse to remove organic debris, soak for 15 to 30 minutes per manufacturer's instructions for tuberculocidal effectiveness, rinse thoroughly with water, air-dry, bag, and store in clean area. Discard solution according to manufacturer's instructions. (*Mycobacterium tuberculosis* is among the most resistant microorganisms and is used as an indicator of the effectiveness of chemical germicides. A tuberculocidal disinfectant is considered high-level.)

Standard disinfection: Clean to remove organic debris before disinfecting. Use a 1:10 solution of household chlorine bleach and water (1 part bleach to 9 parts water) and scrub vigorously with clean cloth material (laundered rags or gauze pads) or use an EPA-registered germicidal/viricidal agent per manufacturer's instructions. Prepare fresh chlorine solution daily. Note that chlorine will cause clouding on plexiglass and corrosion of metal after prolonged use, and will bleach fabrics and carpets if spilled. Aluminum surfaces should be decontaminated with clean cloth material saturated with 70 to 90 percent isopropyl or ethyl alcohol.

Sterilization: Use hospital facilities.

EQUIPMENT/CLEANING LIST

Air Splints: Scrub with hot soapy detergent, rinse with water, and dry before use.

Backboards and straps: Scrub with hot soapy detergent, rinse with water, and dry before use.

Bag mask: Wear gloves. Bag mask should be taken apart, scrubbed in hot soapy water, rinsed, and disinfected by soaking in cold liquid sterilization agent (e.g., glutaraldehyde 1:4 for 30 minutes) after each use. Air dry thoroughly. Follow manufacturer's instructions for use of chemical.

C-collars: Scrub with hot soapy detergent, rinse with water, and dry before use.

Clothing: Clean and disinfect clothing soiled with blood and body fluids by machine washing in 160°F water for 25 minutes. Chlorine bleach provides an extra margin of safety. If low-temperature (below 160°F) household laundry cycles are used, be sure to use bleach. All-fabric bleaches are effective.

Defibrillator and paddles: Clean external plastic surfaces per manufacturer's instructions or with Formula 409 or equivalent.

Intubation equipment: Wear gloves to protect hands. Clean all parts in hot, soapy water to remove organic debris, rinse, and rough dry. Soak laryngoscope blade for 30 minutes in 1:4 glutaraldehyde solution for high-level disinfection. Remove from solution, rinse with water, and dry. Store bagged in clean area. Discard solution according to manufacturer's instructions. Follow standard disinfection procedures for other parts.

KED devices: Scrub with hot soapy detergent, rinse with water, and dry before use.

Linens: See Clothing.

Manikins: CPR training manikins should be cleaned and disinfected during and after classes according to the Centers for Disease Control guidelines. Between students, if individual protective face shields are not used, the manikin face and area inside the mouth should be wiped *vigorously* with clean absorbent material (e.g., 4 in. × 4 in. gauze pad) wet with a solution of ¼ cup bleach per gallon of water. Surfaces should remain wet for at least 30 seconds before they are wiped dry with a second piece of clean absorbent material. After class, manikins should be disassembled, thoroughly washed inside and out with warm, soapy water and brushes, rinsed, and disinfected with bleach solution left on for at least 10 minutes. Disinfection should be followed by a water rinse and thorough drying before storage. An alcohol rinse will aid drying of internal surfaces.

MAST pants: Scrub with hot soapy detergent, rinse with water, and dry *thoroughly* before storing.

O_2 bottle: Scrub with hot soapy detergent, rinse with water, and dry before use.

Penrose tubing: Dispose if possible or scrub with hot soapy detergent, rinse with water, and dry before use. Use liquid disinfectant if contaminated with body fluids.

Splints—metal: Scrub with hot soapy detergent, rinse with water, and dry before use.

Stethoscopes: Wipe after use with alcohol swabs.

Suction equipment: Catheter tips: Discard. Units: should be cleaned after each use. Wear gloves and handle suction secretions with caution. Disposable: Cap and remove liner and tubing, and dispose with potentially infectious waste. Non-disposable: Empty bottle carefully down drain at drain level, disinfect with germicidal, viricidal agent, and air dry. Flush and soak tubing with disinfectant solution and air dry.

Vacuum splints: Scrub with hot soapy detergent, rinse with water, and dry before use.

Vehicle surfaces: Clean with hot soapy water and disinfect work surfaces with a 1:10 chlorine bleach solution or other viricidal agent. Pay special attention to steering wheel and accessories such as radio equipment, spotlight handles, and kit handles that come into contact with the hands. It is good practice to wipe down high-contact work surfaces after every transport, and it is essential to do so after blood/body fluid spills or transport of an infectious patient. Blood/body fluid spills should be cleaned by gloving up, cleaning with soap and water, and disinfecting with fresh 1:10 bleach solution. Large pools of blood should be blotted with paper towels before attempting disinfection. Floors and walls do not have to be disinfected unless they have been exposed to blood or body fluids. Airing is ineffective as a disinfectant.

Waste Disposal

Dispose of all wastes safely. In the EMS setting, potentially infectious waste includes needles and sharps, blood and blood products, secretions, soiled linens, and dressings from infected wounds. To prevent the spread of disease, it is important to dispose of these materials in a safe manner.

Needles and sharps should be deposited in rigid, puncture-proof containers manufactured for this purpose. Dispose syringe with needle. When containers are full, arrange for disposal by a hospital, or according to local health regulations.

Medical disposables that have been exposed to blood or body fluids should be placed in sturdy, leakproof plastic bags (wear gloves!). This waste should be kept in a secure place (e.g., locked dumpster) prior to disposal in a landfill or by arrangement with a hospital with incineration or other infectious waste disposal facilities.

   Dispose of liquefied waste such as suction secretions by holding container at drain level and pouring liquid slowly and carefully down the drain. Flush with water and disinfect container. Disinfect sink with bleach solution. Do *not* pour into storm drains.

Communicable Disease Reference Guide

For a complete description of communicable diseases and prevention and control measures, refer to the most recent edition of *Control of Communicable Diseases in Man* (American Public Health Association). Note that many diseases can be asymptomatic when infectious, or not infectious when symptomatic. Accordingly, care providers should use appropriate protective measures on a routine basis. Wear gloves and other barrier protection as necessary, exercise caution with needles and sharps, use ventilation devices, use good handwashing technique, dispose of wastes safely, and clean and disinfect vehicles and equipment appropriately.

Disease or Condition	Symptoms	Transmission	Protection	Exposure Followup[a]
AIDS, ARC (acquired immune deficiency syndrome; AIDS-related complex)	None; or fever, night sweats, dry cough, weight loss, diarrhea, swollen lymph nodes, skin lesions (painless pink, brown, or purple), persistent or recurrent yeast infections, or other signs of opportunistic infection or cancer.	Sexual contact, shared IV drugs, infection of newborn by mother, blood transfusions before 3/85; in EMS setting, by introduction of blood or body fluid through the skin or by contact with eye, mouth, or nose; no known cases transmitted by saliva	Gloves, protection of broken skin, handwashing; gowns, masks, or eye protection, as necessary for large amounts of blood; ventilation device advised; needles/sharps precautions	For percutaneous exposure of blood, immediately wipe off blood and apply alcohol to wound, wash ASAP; for mucocutaneous exposure, irrigate with water or saline; report to supervisor; document
Chickenpox	Fever, sore throat, skin eruptions that rupture and scab.	Respiratory secretions; or contact with shingles lesions	Gloves, ventilation device, handwashing, (mask)[b]	Varicella zoster immune globulin (VZIG) within 96 hours, for high-risk individuals (e.g., those who have not had chickenpox, newborns, immunocompromised patients); document exposure

164

CMV (cytomegalovirus infection)	Usually none; in infants, severe general infection, 5–10% of newborns have congenital abnormalities, and 10–20% develop them early in life; in adults, symptoms may be fever, swollen lymph glands, rash, sore throat, liver and spleen enlargement; 30–80% of population have antibodies	Percutaneous or mucosal contact with infected semen, blood, cervical secretions, urine, saliva, and breast milk	Gloves, handwashing, ventilation device	Document exposure
Conjunctivitis (pinkeye)	Tearing, irritation, swelling of eyes, discharge	Contact with discharge from upper respiratory tract or eye, usually by contaminated fingers, clothing, shared makeup applicators	Gloves, handwashing, personal hygiene	If contracted, medical treatment with topical ointment; document exposure
Gonorrhea	In men, urethral discharge, and pain on urination; in women, none, or pain on urination, discharge, lower abdominal pain, and frequent urination	Sexual contact, including oral-genital contact, and from mother to infant at birth	Gloves, handwashing	If exposure, testing and appropriate treatment (antibiotics may be prescribed); document exposure
Hepatitis A	Fever, loss of appetite, fatigue, nausea, abdominal pain, jaundice, light-colored stool, dark-colored urine	Contact with stool or blood of infected person; contaminated food or water	Gloves, handwashing	If ingestion, immunization with immune globulin (IG) ASAP within 2 weeks; document exposure

Disease or Condition	Symptoms	Transmission	Protection	Exposure Followup[a]
Hepatitis B	Nausea and vomiting, loss of appetite, sometimes fever, abdominal discomfort, sometimes jaundice, diarrhea	Sexual contact, shared IV drugs, from mother at birth; in EMS setting, by blood-to-blood, or mucous membrane exposure to blood or body fluids	Immunization + gloves, handwashing, ventilation device, needles/sharps precautions	Depending on antibody status, vaccine and immune globulin may be indicated; document exposure
Herpes simplex types 1 and 2 (cold sore, fever blister, blister-like genital lesions)	Itching, tingling sensation, followed by lesion(s); sometimes asymptomatic	Mucous membrane contact with lesion, or through break in skin; sexual contact with lesions, from mother to infant at birth	Gloves, handwashing, ventilation device if oral lesions present	Document exposure
Herpetic whitlow (from herpesvirus type 1 or 2, or zoster)	Pain, swelling, redness of fingers, nerve impairment	Contact with herpesvirus through a break in the skin	Gloves, handwashing	Document exposure
Herpes zoster (shingles)	Painful, itching lesions	Reactivation of dormant chickenpox virus; contact with lesions can cause chickenpox in those without immunity	Gloves, handwashing	Document exposure; zoster immune globulin may be indicated for susceptible adults
Influenza	Fever, chills, headache, fatigue, sore throat, cough, muscle aches, runny nose	Respiratory droplets; virus lives for hours in dried mucus	Annual immunization, gloves, handwashing, (mask[b])	Amantadine administered early in type A disease reduces symptoms; document exposure

Lice	Itching, visible eggs on hair, clothing	Close personal contact; sharing of personal items; pubic lice (crabs) by sexual contact, from bedding, clothing	Gloves	Document exposure; wash exposed clothing in hot water; if infested, use appropriate medicated soap
Measles	Fever, conjunctivitis, runny nose, cough, Koplik's spots (small, irregular bright red spots, with a bluish-white speck in the center of each, inside the cheek), red, blotchy skin rash; most common among preschool children, adolescents, young adults	Respiratory droplets, direct contact with nasal and throat secretions, and less commonly, by contact with items soiled with such secretions	Immunization, gloves, handwashing, (mask[b])	Document exposure
Meningitis (bacterial)	Fever, nausea, often vomiting, intense headache, stiff neck, rash on lower part of body; Affects young children; uncommon in adults over 25; asymptomatic carriers	Direct contact with discharges from nose and throat	Ventilation device, gloves, handwashing, (mask[b])	If preventive measures not followed, and suction, intubation, or ventilation involved; ampicillin or rifampin may be prescribed; document exposure
Meningitis (viral or aseptic)	Stiff neck and back, headache, fever, sore throat, nausea, drowsiness, sometimes abdominal or chest pains, rash	Contact with infected feces	Gloves, handwashing, (mask[b])	No drug therapy; active disease rarely exceeds 10 days; document exposure

167

Disease or Condition	Symptoms	Transmission	Protection	Exposure Followup[a]
Mononucleosis	Fever, sore throat, swollen lymph glands (posterior cervical), fatigue	Direct contact with saliva	Ventilation device, gloves, handwashing	Document exposure
Mumps	Fever, swelling, and tenderness of one or more salivary glands; inflammation of the testes or ovaries in those past puberty; more common in older children	Respiratory droplets, contact with saliva	Immunization, ventilation device, gloves, handwashing, (mask[b])	Document exposure
Pertussis (whooping cough)	Repeated violent coughs, without inhalation, followed by a whooping sound; usually a disease of young children	Respiratory droplets	Ventilation device, gloves, handwashing, immunization before age 7, (mask[b])	Document exposure; antibiotics may be indicated
Pneumonia (bacterial)	Chills, fever, pain in lungs, difficulty breathing, cough producing rusty sputum	Respiratory droplets, direct oral contact, contact with items soiled with respiratory discharges	Ventilation device, gloves, handwashing, (mask[b])	Document exposure; antibiotics may be indicated
Rabies	Feeling of apprehension, headache, fever, malaise; later, paralysis, delirium, convulsions	Direct contact with saliva of infected animal, usually by bite, sometimes through break in skin or intact mucous membrane; no documented human-to-human transmission	Ventilation device, gloves, handwashing	Document exposure; wash animal bite thoroughly; tetanus, rabies immune globulin, and rabies vaccine, as indicated

Rubella (German measles)	Fever, headache, mild rash, conjunctivitis, swollen glands behind ears and at base of skull	Respiratory droplets, contact with nasopharyngeal secretions, blood, urine, stool, from mother to fetus	Immunization, ventilation device, gloves, handwashing, (mask[b])	Document exposure
Scabies	Itchy lesions, usually on finger folds, breasts, abdomen, lower buttocks, inside elbows and wrists; lesions are burrows of a tiny mite	Skin-to-skin contact	Gloves, handwashing	Document exposure; treat with medicated lotion
Syphilis	Phase 1: painless lesion, anywhere on body; phase 2: may include enlarged lymph nodes, reddish rash on palms of hands/soles of feet, fever, headache, sore throat, loss of appetite; phase 3: none	Sexual contact, blood	Gloves, handwashing; needles/sharps precautions	Document exposure; testing and treatment may be indicated
Tuberculosis	May include productive cough, fever, night sweats, coughing up blood, weakness	Airborn droplets, prolonged contact	Ventilation device, gloves, handwashing, (mask[b])	Document exposure

[a] Maintain accurate records of exposures (needlesticks, blood/body fluid: mucous membrane contact) to ensure adequate follow-up and record keeping for Workers' Compensation purposes.
[b] Masks are not recommended for routine use. If patient is known to have a disease transmitted by respiratory secretions and the care provider does not have immunity, the patient may be masked to protect the care provider. The risk of airborne transmission of communicable diseases is low unless mouth-to-mouth is performed.

APPENDIX 18: SYRUP OF IPECAC

DEFINITION

This drug is given to cause a person to vomit.

ADMINISTERING THE DRUG

It is given to patients who have ingested poisons or have taken an overdose of medication. EMS services require an order from a physician or poison control center before the EMT gives this medication.

DO NOT give ipecac to the following patients:

1. With signs of decreased level of consciousness
2. Pregnant women
3. With a history of heart or esophageal disease
4. Has had a seizure due to the poisoning or overdose
5. Has ingested strong acids or alkali products, or caustic substances
6. Has ingested petroleum products (the poison control center may advise otherwise on recently ingested petroleum products)

Dosage

Adults and children over age 12: 2 tablespoons or 30 mL
Children 1 to 12 years old: 1 tablespoon or 15 mL
Infants less than 1 year old: 2 teaspoons or 10 mL

PATIENT CARE

1. After the patient has swallowed the ipecac, give him two to four 8-ounce glasses of water or carbonated soft drink, or the amount specified by the poison control center.
2. Position the person to prevent aspiration while vomiting.
3. Transport the patient as soon as possible.

4. If the patient does not vomit in approximately 20 minutes, you may be asked to give a second dose.
5. Save all emesis and transport it with the patient.

SPECIAL CONSIDERATIONS

All persons to whom the EMT has given ipecac must be transported to an emergency facility. If patients do not vomit following ipecac ingestion, it must be removed from their stomachs.